AGAINST THE GRAIN

Free Yourself From Flour and Lose Weight Permanently

- *Say Goodbye to that Dysfunctional Union!*
- *Overcome a 'Battered' Relationship with Food!*
- *End the Cycle Of LOATHE, LOSE, GAIN, REPEAT!*
- *Enjoy Delicious, Guilt-Free Eating!*

Sandy Thompson, EYYO, PT
(ex yo-yo dieter, permanently thin)

With Ellen Singer

authorHOUSE™

1663 LIBERTY DRIVE, SUITE 200
BLOOMINGTON, INDIANA 47403
(800) 839-8640
WWW.AUTHORHOUSE.COM

First published by AuthorHouse 03/09/05

ISBN: 1-4208-1960-7 (sc)

Library of Congress Control Number: 2004195068

Printed in the United States of America
Bloomington, Indiana

This book is printed on acid-free paper.

"Before starting any diet or exercise program, we recommend consulting your healthcare professional."

This book is dedicated to you, and your desire to make a change.

You go girl!

Acknowledgements

Cindy – you are so deeply imbedded in my heart. Your generosity is astounding, and so is your talent. This book could not have happened without you, and you know why!

And Cheryl, thank you for your unwavering support for my vision, and for sharing some pretty meaty belly laughs.

Jen, without your technical perspective, I'd still be writing. You rock!

My gorgeous daughter, Janna, you are my entire inspiration. My hero. Even though it hasn't always been easy being my daughter, you make me feel like I am the best Mom (and woman) in the world. I love you.

And to my family, Mom, Dad, Elaine & Peter… thanks for sharing my passions, even when it was all about me.

Ellen, you helped me share my voice with such eloquence and humor. I believe I chose the best.

And to my extraordinary, handsome and sweet husband Paul. I love you for believing in me in a way that most women only dream of.

Introduction

"Inside me lives a skinny woman crying to get out.
But I can usually shut the bitch up with cookies."

—Unknown

This was the story of my life. And I presume yours too if you are reading this book....

How long have you been dieting?

Since you stopped fitting into your pre-pregnancy clothes?

Since the invention of Spandex? Since you had to record (and lie about) your weight on your driver's license? Since the very first time you filled out a driver's license application – fifteen, twenty, thirty years ago?

In other words, have you been dieting forever? And feeling guilty, inadequate and maybe even hopeless because you're not getting any thinner – and maybe fatter! – Or because your weight fluctuates more often than the price of gasoline?

Isn't it time to stop? Stop dieting, and find a real solution and a new path toward PERMANENT weight maintenance.

I found that path and it's simple (not easy, magical or miraculous), and it works for women with the lifestyle, time constraints, responsibilities and stresses that most of us share. Women like you. Women like me.

When I stopped dieting seven years ago and started listening to what my body was telling me, I lost – and kept off – weight for the first time in my adult life.

And you can do it, too. Because when it comes to knowing what eating patterns work for you, YOU are the expert. You know which foods satisfy you, which ones make you hungrier, which ones trigger eating binges that incite you to raid the 7-11 snack aisle at ten at night.

You KNOW but again, if you're like me, your desperation to be thin overrode your common sense and you've been had by every fad diet and burnt by every fat-burning pill on the market.

Why have people been telling you to count calories, eliminate fat and/or carbs when the evidence – your tummy, hips and thighs – proves that none of these methods works in maintaining your desired weight?

Because a lot of people have been getting rich off of your misery. Some 129.6 million overweight Americans have spent nearly $33 billion annually to find the answer to permanent weight loss and good health, but the answers we get are more often borne of corporate greed than our dietary needs.

Thanks to the wonders of marketing, even doctors (who should really know better) fell victim to one of the greatest and longest lasting hoaxes of the twentieth century: the low-fat, high-carbohydrate diet. Now, with equal enthusiasm, but no greater examination, many are leaping on the new -- and, perhaps polar-opposite low-carb trend.

Just like most of us, the medical community has been prey to the manipulations of the marketing departments at Quaker Oatmeal, Kellogg's and now Atkin's, and EVERY brand that stood to gain market share by creating the great American diet trends -- from fat-hating to grain-loving to carb-avoiding mania.

How can I be so sure?

Because I've been a marketer for most of my professional life, and I know how we pounce on every trend we like, ignore any that don't serve us, and invent trends when it profits us to do so.

As a former public relations executive for a national retail chain, I was responsible for building sales with a back-to-school marketing campaign. I had nothing to work with. It wasn't the year of short hem lines, baggy shirts, boot-cut jeans or black everything. It was a year in which kid's fashion had an undefined 'anything goes' attitude, and the excitement of back-to-school shopping was becoming a thing of the past.

What I needed was a trend, so I created one. I decided that the best way to generate buzz was to tie fashion into the emerging focus on cultural diversity and proclaim it the 'Year of Individuality'. I had to back up that claim (advertisers can make that leap; PR people must ground their proclamations in research); so I devised a questionnaire, framing the questions in such a way that the answers were pretty much guaranteed to support my "theory". I manipulated the survey questions so that self expression and individuality would be what school age children wanted.

It worked! Individuality was the news in Back-to-School fashion, and with an aggressive PR campaign, I was invited on several talk shows to discuss the trends and promote the fact that choice, individuality and value are what our stores could give kids and their parents.

Do I KNOW that aggressive marketing is why we are a nation of 135 million fatties – growing in number and pant size yearly? No I don't, and it's not the goal of this book to try. Rather, it's to give you reason to question everything you've ever read about weight loss and maintenance so that you can become your own weight loss guru.

That's what I did seven years ago. After years of gaining and losing hundreds of pounds (twenty off, thirty on, give or take ten each round), I finally decided to stop believing the hype (what took me so long?) and trust my own intuition.

I had read (and continue to read) diet books, magazines and medical journals, but like so many women hungry for a quick-fix to a lifelong struggle with weight, I only absorbed what I wanted to hear.

This was 1997. We were universally passing the pasta and passing on Dr. Atkins. (His recent glorification in some circles was several New Year's resolutions away). I had no idea what would work to help me attain – and maintain – a healthy weight. All I knew is that nothing I'd tried to date had worked.

Not exactly true. I'd been able to lose weight on any diet I tried – and I tried practically all of them – but I could NEVER maintain the weight loss. So I re-examined the theories again, this time with a more critical eye, and I also took a more objective look at my relationship with food.

What food did I love the most? No doubt, it was bread, pasta, cookies & bagels. What food did I most often crave? Bread, pasta, cookies & bagels. What food did I most often overeat, stuffing myself after both cravings and hunger had been satisfied? Bread, pasta, bagels…

Grains were good for America – that's what the experts said – but maybe, just maybe, grains weren't good for me.

And that's how I started on my FINAL weight loss journey. By going *Against the Grain* of both popular wisdom and my Italian-American heritage, I began to solve the riddle of my own weight problem.

One simple philosophy and three short words – NO MORE FLOUR – did for me what no other diet theory or plan ever did –slip into size six jeans for the past seven years without being hungry, without temptation and nasty cravings, and without feeling deprived!

Against the Grain describes my struggle and my victory over deeply-rooted weight and self-esteem issues and shows you how you can become master of your own health and fitness destiny. Eliminating flour gave me fantastic freedom that I want you to realize and embrace. It eliminates the fear and guilt of watching, worrying -- and regretting what I put into my mouth as long as I avoid all grains. I'm not perfect -- I do slip up occasionally (eat too many nuts here, a few extra chunks of low-fat cheese there). But as long as the food I'm overeating DOES NOT include grains, I am confident I will not return to old weight-gaining habits. We'll discuss the WHY of this later in the book, but trust me on this, there is enormous freedom, incredible power when you say no to flour.

My research and my seven years of success support the no-grain philosophy, and I will be an avid proponent of its benefits. But I believe that every woman knows her body best and if you heed that understanding and combine it with available evidence, you will find weight management success whether your solution is the same, slightly dissimilar or completely opposite of mine.

I've done the research, so you don't have to. *Against the Grain* will be the *Reader's Digest* version of what's been written about weight loss in the past fifteen years. If you want to know the foundation of the three most popular diet camps – low-fat, low-carb and the Hollywood elitist raw diet – you'll find it in *Against the Grain*. If you want to know what the genesis of the Scarsdale Diet, which led to the Atkins Diet, which led to the Pritikin Diet, Zone Diet, which led to the South Beach, and Dr. Phil diets -- and then back to Dr. Atkin's again -- you'll find it in *Against the Grain*. (And don't forget the diets your mother/sister/doctor/hairdresser told you about!) *Against the Grain* gives the facts you need to know so that you can separate them from the fiction you may have learned.

And why should any woman, feeling fat and frustrated and wary of being sucked in again – listen to me?

Because I am that woman. I survived being that woman, and broke through the mind set that kept me trapped inside a plump woman's body even when my jeans were loose-fitting. I survived being the woman who tried every fad diet on the market *knowing* they were destined to fail (the Grapefruit Diet? Come on!) I survived being that woman who felt uncomfortable, unloved and undeserving no matter what I accomplished or who I was with – because my waistline was my only barometer of self worth. I survived being that woman who believed she failed every diet she tried even when logic told her that the diet had failed her.

I survived being a miserable, chubby woman in America. And my mission is to help other women like me become survivors too.

I am not a guru. I do not promise easy answers.

But I promise to help you find the answers you can live with – as a healthy, lean woman – for the rest of your life. And I promise to encourage and inspire you every step of the way.

I'll also introduce you to Ellen, who's just begun her weight-management journey. Her story mirrors mine with a twist. She was thin for most of the years I was heavy by following her natural inclinations for a protein-rich diet, then got fat when she adopted a "heart-smart diet" and fatter still EVERY time she stripped a little more meat and cholesterol from her diet. Since talking to me and devising her own plan, she's lost thirty of the fifty pounds she couldn't lose for ten years!

Against the Grain is written for and by women who share the same pains, the same gains and, I hope, the same losses of a lifetime.

Table of Contents

Part One:

Saying Goodbye to a Dysfunctional (food) Relationship

Chapter One:
Grain of Hope

If you're like me, you've been on more diets than dates and had your heart (and scales) repeatedly broken by the same scoundrels such as Cal Counters, Will Power and Lowe Phatt. But as a true glutton (for punishment), you keep falling for the latest Great Weight Hope and setting yourself up for one food relationship disaster after another.

Maybe you still hang on to the tools, hoping that some day they will be your key to permanent weight loss... serrated spoons from the Grapefruit Diet, chopsticks from the Rice Diet, a blender from the Liquid Diet, a faucet filter from the Water Diet. And still, the unwanted pounds hang onto you.

You've chewed the fat with Dr. Atkins and eschewed it with Dr. Pritikin. You've zoned in and out of diets from Scarsdale to Beverly Hills. You've practiced hypnosis and ketosis to the point of neurosis and experienced the highs and lows of fat and carbohydrate mania. You're pushing – or past—forty and you're feeling anything but Fit & Fabulous.

Some days you joke in the office that you're a size four – squared – but most nights you look at your rounded belly and sigh. And if no one's looking, you cry.

Being an overweight woman in America has much less to do with what clothes fit than it does with fitting in. No matter what our social or financial status, whether our income is six figures or four – it's our dress size that determines the size of our self-esteem. For most of my life, the labels on my clothes and the labels on my forehead bounced around in opposite directions. When I could zip up a pair of size six jeans, I was Confident, Sexy and Powerful. When I was struggling with the buttons on a pair of size fourteen khakis, I was Lazy, Weak and Undesirable. Maybe I needed therapy more than I needed a diet plan but I don't think it would have put me any closer to my desired weight. We are who we look like, it's part of the female psyche. There's no logic in the assumption that Fat equals Lazy. Anyone who's ever struggled with her weight knows that it's easier to *be* slim than fat, and it's not even an unbearable burden to *get* slim. It's *staying,* slim that seems impossible, and we blame ourselves each time we fail.

It only took me about thirty-five years, and as many diets, to consider the possibility that the fault wasn't mine, that maybe there was something wrong with the diets. That theory absolved me of some guilt, but it didn't solve my problem. If what I needed was a different diet, how and where would I find it? Did I wait for the next diet guru to tell me THE answer, or did I solve this problem the way I'd solved every other in my life – from my gut? Really, what was I thinking? I didn't listen to my mother when she advised me to learn a practical profession (not ill advice considering I was an unwed, teenage welfare mom). No, I went to acting school instead, a decision that saved my life. So why couldn't I save my figure from being identified by my rather large ass?

Well, I could and did seven years ago. By going *Against the Grain*, I lost forty pounds and have kept them off without hunger and without sacrifice. I'm happy, healthy and still fit into the size six jeans I bought in 1997. I'll tell you how later but let me first tell you how I became a plump child, a fatter adolescent and a yo-yo dieter for twenty-five years.

I wasn't born to be fat – but it was the center of my identity ever since I can remember.

Dinner in my Italian-American home consisted of equal, heaping portions of pasta, bread and guilt, and I dove in headfirst for seconds of everything.

Maybe your fat path was strewn with different food-emotion combos. But I'm guessing you got there in pretty much the same way – some unhealthy mix of calories and criticism served from morning 'til bedtime – that burdened you with a less than ideal body and far from healthy self image.

Bad eating habits and poor self-esteem are hard to break away from. Instead, they grow into dysfunctional relationships – like the love-hate relationship I had with both food and my family – designed to last a lifetime.

It's a story we all share. It's typical. Predictable. Textbook.

Food was the love and praise I craved. When its powers waned – when a plate of lasagna couldn't make up for the praises of my parents– I sought physical and emotional comfort elsewhere. I found it with a boy whose testosterone kept pace with my neediness. We both ignored the likely outcome of this match-up until our irresponsibility was rewarded with new hormones and new needs – I became pregnant at age seventeen. (I thought I was fat before the pregnancy. Boy, did I have a lot of surprises in store over the next forty weeks and beyond!)

One bad mistake deserves another. I married the boy.

It's what my parents wanted me to do, it's what I believed I owed them. I ignored my own doubts – the father was as immature as I was – and caved to the familiar and familial pressures to "do the right thing."

There was no fairy tale ending to our story. Just the sad realities of mixing a boy, a girl and a baby in an unwanted alliance.

I was divorced at 19.

This was my second major failure in less than two years, and I was about to add a third, welfare. The price of accepting public assistance was tolerating both public and private humiliation. My family and the neighborhood were quick to remind me of my mediocrity. But the worst criticism – the self-loathing, self-doubt and increasing sense of isolation – was self-inflicted punishment, and no one was crueler to me than I was. How did I comfort – and torment – myself at the same time? Not another man, thank you, just lots of raviolis.

I gained weight, hid beneath sweaters and long jackets, and essentially punished myself for the single crime of being the lead character in my own life's story. The story of a VICTIM! I had a screaming red V pasted to my chest, and I was about to collect a few more letters in my loser's alphabet.

At age 20, I was diagnosed with Grave's Disease – a debilitating auto-immune condition of the thyroid gland, which throws your body into a frenzy of heart palpitations, hot flashes, metabolic fluctuations and head-to-toe tremors. I had extreme weight loss before it was diagnosed but once they got it under control, I was just my old fat self. It takes awhile for thyroid supplements to compensate for the loss of the natural hormone. It took even longer for someone like me to recover from what seemed another failure. I was still living at home (C is for controlling mother), still collecting welfare, (W is for Worthless) and still figuring out how to care for a two-year-old daughter (S is for Stupid). Was this as good as it gets? (R is for Resigned) Would it only get worse? (D is for Depressed)

Thank God there are only twenty-six letters in the alphabet. If only there were a finite number of excuses we could give ourselves for not accomplishing our goals, maybe we'd reach them.

In the midst of this misery, it occurred to me that I'd been sidetracked from answering a child's most-oft-asked question: What do you want to be when you grow up?

I'd allowed the question to be answered for me – first by an unplanned pregnancy, then by parents who told me what I *should* do – live at home, go to state college, learn a good 'trade'.

I didn't buy it, thank God! Instead, at a time when it seemed I had nothing going for me, I found the courage to follow my heart rather than hide behind my poor self-image.

I packed up my daughter and all of our belongings and drove off across the country for Pasadena, CA to enroll in a school for the performing arts. Everybody thought I must have lost my mind. Breaking away from the security of my family at such a low point in my life was widely regarded as an unusual way to secure a better future.

It saved my life, shaped my career, and eventually led me to solve my biggest struggle – weight and, consequently, my self-image – in the same way.

I never became a professional performing artist. That wasn't the point. I learned what I could do, what I could accomplish when I believed in my own instincts, my own strengths.

In every instance, the results have been powerful and lasting; and, in every instance, the results have come because I have dared to defy conventional wisdom by jumping way out of the box to fulfillment.

I want to share my experiences with you, help you define your own box, then show you how to lift yourself out of it and into the body (and mind) that fits you best.

I have come to know for certain that wherever you are in life, you don't have to stay there. It's simply a matter of deciding you aren't going to be bounced around inside life's big, noisy pinball machine like a little silver nothing.

You – nobody else - choose your lifestyle, commitments and relationships. I believe that the body you have is the body you choose. It has less to do with luck, genes and desire to be thin than it does with the choices you are making on a daily basis.

You can choose– right here, right now to win your last war on weight by embracing the *Against the Grain* philosophy. Regardless of the circumstances you face or the failures you've endured, you can reclaim your spirit, your passion and your purpose, and, ultimately, be at peace with your weight.

So let's get busy.

Chapter Two:
A Grain of Truth, A Pound of Lies

If losing weight is so easy, fast and guaranteed, then why are half of all Americans still overweight? Why does obesity, now officially declared an epidemic, remain a mystery as to both cause and solution? How could the doctors, scientists and nutritionists (not to mention the cereal and pasta companies) be so certain (and yet maybe so wrong) about carbohydrates and fat? How can Dr. Atkins be a hero, villain and hero again from one decade to the next? His message is pretty much the same. And if a pH-balanced, vegetable rich diet is THE solution to fitness and wellness, then why isn't every wheat-grass-drinking vegetarian forever thin?

The diet and health experts – who tell us the what, when, where, and how to lose weight and then maintain it – simply can't understand the most important part of sustained weight control: YOU.

You are the great, unscientific variable in their purportedly scientific programs. You are the wildcard in every painfully hyped diet, regimen and program. Until you conquer it yourself, there is no program on the planet that will work. Period.

In the end, you are the one who makes the difference. And you are the one who keeps paying the pound of flesh for programs that work for a while then collapse because their "solutions" are simply unbearable over the long run. Worst of all, many of these programs are also flat-out unhealthy.

I know because I spent the first thirty-five years of my life being alternately charmed and victimized by every diet-du-jour and self-hyped weight loss guru.

So what, you ask, makes me any different? How can Sandy Somebody produce a weight-loss solution that has evaded so-called experts forever without all the usual credentials that would make her qualified?

Because I've lived through the pains and gains, made the mistakes, had the setbacks and finally overcame my struggle with weight maintenance. Now I want to pass on that knowledge and experience to help others avoid those same mistakes. **This makes me a true expert in what I am writing about!**

My proof is in the scales. My proof is in my struggle. My proof is in your frustrations, your hopes – high, dashed and renewed many times over – and the belief that your weight controls you, identifies you and limits you.

My success didn't come easy. Like you, I lived the endless cycle of loathe-lose-gain-repeat. I spent and sweated and ate every diet food from egg whites to flavored cardboard. Several years ago, I finally broke out of the endless loop of feeling thin today and fat tomorrow. I did it by creating my own battle-plan based on equal parts of science, insight, intuition and hard-earned experience.

Now I feel committed to helping you –women with a similar decades-old struggle -- discover and leverage the same basic principles I used to finally achieve a permanent, healthy (and easy to clothe) body weight.

What makes me different? First of all, I'm not a guru, I'm a survivor. Secondly, I will tell you the truth from my experience, not my business plan. I will share and interpret all the scientific malarkey based on my experiences. Rather than trying to get rich quick with another breakthrough concept that won't work, I will put all of my energy into helping you get healthy with practical ideas, strategies and inspiration.

This demands one essential commitment on your part: you must be willing to inwardly challenge all of the experts by listening to and learning from your own body, mind and spirit.

It will be your responsibility to take even the most educated opinions and balance them against the wisdom of the real authority on this subject: YOU. After all, you're the make or break element in this equation and you will be the one who decides whether or not you want to and will be slim.

You've most likely walked enough miles on the treadmill to end up in China, right? And you've blown thousands of dollars on special foods and lean, mean diet machines.

What have you learned? Plenty? What have you gained? Most likely, weight. Me, too. But several years ago, I finally put an end to it all – and this book is the result.

One thing I learned is that those gurus know as much or more about marketing and chemistry than they do about you, me or the misery and discomfort of being overweight.

True, chemistry is the gritty stuff that explains how matter (food) transforms (chemical reactions) into other matter (more food) that makes us fat. It's also the perplexing nonsense that muddies the waters with contradictions about good foods and bad foods, protein intake, carb intake, calorie counting and water weight.

Another thing I learned is that they'd rather see you buy their products than see you through to permanent weight maintenance. That's where the marketing comes in…that's the stuff that persuades us to buy everything from Cocoa Puffs to OxyClean whether we need it or not. It is the marketers right and responsibility to share their news and views with consumers, but the manipulating spin has gotten out of hand in the diet industry.

Now it's time to shake loose from established claims and formulate our own success strategies. That's what's so useful about this book: it's loaded with independent interpretations of all kinds of information I have gathered, sorted and culled over the years. But every element of it – from the thinking, learning, planning and doing – will be performed by you.

I make you this promise: I will tell you what I think and never proclaim it to be gospel or guaranteed. Why? Because I know for a fact that everyone's body is different…and that, more importantly, everyone's commitment to health (and relationship with food) is unique.

I'll promise you something else, too: you'll never see my abs doing contortions on TV. Why? Because my abs are flat -- not ripped. And my 40-something arms look really good -- but they aren't going to win me any body-building contests. Unlike the hard bodies pushing everything from powders to pills, I am an inquisitive, independent person who simply got tired of being manipulated by the "This is THE Answer" diet industry.

Do you really want veins popping out of your biceps and quads that twitch when you walk? Wouldn't you just rather look and feel great by *your* standards?

Your weight loss – and weight maintenance program – is about YOU – not about me and certainly not about THEM – the doctors and the experts, their promises or programs. When you realize this – as I finally did seven years ago, you eliminate all the ridiculous noise and confusion. When you realize this – as I finally did – you will also end your abdication of responsibility for your own health and well-being.

Against the Grain is a **simple plan** to help you fight through the nonsense and begin to win **your** war with **your** weight and, more important, be at permanent peace with your body.

Yes, there are diet recommendations – but they will come with rationale, practical reasons for why they will work and how you can make them a habitual part of your life.

I will describe in detail MY weight management experience and tell you how and why you may want to make it yours.

Here's what I did:
- I totally eliminated flour from my diet.
- I decreased my intake of refined sugar.
- I made sensible choices about fat and dairy.

Now, before you let that self-defeatist message enter your mind and spit out your mouth that you could NEVER give up bread and pasta (just as I did way back) listen with an open mind how it works for me and remember: I am you. I was where you are now. I didn't think I could live without flour. But I made the choice to be thin. I wanted that more than I wanted bread.

But guess what? I was happy without it. I'm still happy without it. And I'm confident you will be happy without it, too. I never let myself go hungry, never feel deprived, and never feel like cheating my commitment. And I don't gain weight.

And after years of losing and gaining the same forty pounds, of never feeling satisfied (either because of hunger or because of the way I looked) of never looking inside a closet that wasn't stocked with both "thin" and "fat" clothes, this is amazing!

So I can say that I am healthy and as lean as is comfortable by my standards– and feeling fabulous.

Why did this program work for me?
- Flour-based foods like bread, pasta and other high carbohydrate foods, such as starchy vegetables and legumes, make me (and probably you) fat so dumping them eliminated the key trigger to **my** weight gain.
- Once I kicked the flour habit, I found that my life-long cravings for these foods evaporated.
- The resulting weight-loss and energy up-tick inspired me to keep going and going to the point where these healthy habits had literally become ingrained in my lifestyle.

After all the painful years of gaining and losing hundreds of pounds, going *Against the Grain* finally enabled me to lose the excess weight and keep it off permanently. The end.

I did it on my own – by my own rules, regulations and dietary restrictions. It freed me from manipulative misinformation. I did it by recognizing that it wasn't the diet or the program that would lose (and keep off) the weight. Losing weight forever was something I would have to do -- and did.

You can do it too.
Without being miserable.

Let's face it: any diet will work if you stick to it and don't die before you reach your goal weight. Can you lose weight drinking milk shakes? Yes! Can I lose weight eating, say, bacon and sausage all the time? Yep. Want to lose weight with fast food! You can. Corn flakes? Sure. Seaweed? I dare you.

But with every diet-regimen we risk two scary things:
- Dying from a horrendously unbalanced diet
- Dying from never-ending boredom

Against the Grain is all about making decisions based on your unique needs, experiences and expectations. It's about tossing all the hype and replacing it with practical, considered common sense.

YOU need to go *Against the Grain* and cut your own path to better health, happiness and well-being. And I intend to help you do just that. I believe the wisdom and lessons in this book will enable you to finally extinguish the self-loathing and ignite your self-confidence.

The diet gurus know they can make you lose ten pounds in two weeks because anybody can do that. What they don't know is that confused and overwhelmed dieters like us need more personalized, permanent solutions to achieve lasting success.

I believe that's what I've found…and I believe that you will find it too.

It's time to find out how. Turn the page.

Chapter Three:
Grain Gain — Ellen's Story

Unlike Sandy, I've only been on two diets in my life.

On the first diet, I lost forty pounds and kept it off for twenty years.

On the second, I *gained* fifty and kept it *on* for more than a decade.

Guess which one was a widely criticized fad diet and which was approved by my doctors and the American Heart Association?

Let me explain how I got thin by doing everything wrong and fat by doing everything right and why I embrace Sandy's going-against-the-grain philosophy.

In 1970, I was 13 and in the eighth grade at a Detroit suburban junior high school. I was taking a required home-economics course in which the assignment was to sew a pair of bell-bottom pants and vest.

This wasn't so horrible. I'd been making my own clothes for a couple of years and had slip-stitched and zig-zagged my way through earlier assignments – an apron, half-slip and patchwork quilt – without putting my seam ripper into use.

But this new project was the first *fitted* outfit, and the teacher made each of pair off and take each other's measurements – in class.

My partner, a hard-edged smoker with a biker boyfriend, was embarrassed by her measurements. They were so tiny the teacher said she'd have to buy a pattern in a child's size eight.

On the other side of the tape measure, my numbers added up to triple digits, and I was instructed – *in front of the entire class* – to purchase my palazzo pants pattern in a size fourteen.

I made the pants and matching vest in a pink-and-green-striped cotton and vowed they'd be too big on me by the time I finished hemming them. I would not, *could no*t be a size fourteen (I'd been squeezing into size twelves just fine, thank you) and I was determined to prove the teacher – and those damning numbers – wrong.

I had a two-part plan: the first was to go on a diet and the second was to narrow my seams from five-eighths to one-half inch (and to take wide turns with the scissors when cutting the material).

Six weeks later, when it was time to try on my new outfit in front of the class, I had to hold up the pants with both hands to keep them from falling off. The teacher was disappointed in me – the pants looked ridiculous – and I was thoroughly relieved. I hung the pants and vest in my closet and kept them there for six years, never wearing them except to occasionally try them on as a reminder of the size fourteen girl I'd *almost* become.

Meanwhile, I was following with religious fervor a popular diet of that decade: The Water Diet. I drank twelve glasses of water a day – four more than the diet mandated – and filled my shrinking tummy with the high-protein fare allowed. I believe I was allowed two condiments – ketchup and horseradish – as well as eggs, meat and cottage cheese. That was about it.

I deviled eggs with the ketchup and horseradish for breakfast, boiled hot dogs and served them with cottage cheese for lunch and ate whatever meat my mother prepared for dinner, removing the skin from chicken and the buns from burgers.

And that was it. I'd never heard of Dr. Atkins at the time and knew nothing of the protein-carbohydrate debate. All I knew is that it worked and by the time the summer rolled around, I stepped on the scales and weighed 108 pounds.

Bye-bye, fat girl! I took my new measurements – 34-23-34 – and threw away all of my old clothes except for the pink pants.

For the next two decades – before, between and after two pregnancies – I kept myself in sizes sixes and eights with minimal exercise and no dieting. My workout routine included sit-ups, stretches and ten minutes on a stationary bike three times a week.

My diet included meat with every meal – I bought steaks by the dozen – a lot of fresh vegetables, small amounts of bread and pastas and from-scratch desserts. Some months, my size six dresses were loose in the waist; others my size eight wool gabardines pulled a bit snugly across my bottom. But even with butter on my breadsticks and forty-pound weight gains with each of pregnancies, at age thirty-five, I was still able to fit into the jeans I bought my first year at the University of Michigan.

Some days I still felt like the fat girl whose thighs rubbed holes in her tights and whose tummy was always bigger than her breasts – bad body images are a lot harder to shed than pounds – but I knew my old Levi's didn't lie.

Then, in the late 1980s, I started to worry about my meat and fat consumption. At cocktail parties, people quoted their cholesterol levels and the Dow Jones average in the same breath. Hosts started calling celery and carrot sticks "crudites" and serving them with fat-free dips. Just try to find a piece of cheese, sausage or corned beef on a deli tray! – if you didn't like turkey – smoked or honeyed – you were out of luck until dessert. Oat bran muffins anyone?

I was a mother now, and I felt an obligation to stay healthy and set a good dietary example for my young daughters. I stopped putting butter (or margarine) on the table, purchased only whole-grain breads, and filled my pantry with black beans, brown rice and yellow corn (to be popped in an air popper and topped with butter-flavored powder) I took eggs and meat off the menu, and the only sweet snacks my girls ate were oatmeal cookies and apple crisp.

I started gaining weight.

By then I KNEW that only fat could make you fat (I read the books, I saw the commercials!), so I found more ways to reduce cholesterol and fat from my diet.

I banned cold cuts, bacon and hot dogs from the house. I removed the skin from chicken before cooking it (didn't want any of that fat seeping into the breast meat) and learned to eat baked potatoes without sour cream, eggs without yolks and meatballs without meat (it was spaghetti and turkey balls for us).

And I gained more weight. My size ten jeans were getting tight, and my none-too-endearing husband was calling me "fat ass."

I was doing everything right, I told myself. Maybe I just needed to be more stringent. I'd had my cholesterol tested for the first time in 1990, and it was so low my doctor told me I could eat a dozen eggs a day without worry (but I'd never do that!). I reasoned, though, that I also didn't need to worry about keeping "good cholesterol" in my diet and since fat was the diet-busting culprit, I'd just get rid of all fat, good or bad. I gave up fish, replaced oil with applesauce in baked goods, and used broth rather than olive oil to saute chicken.

I gained more weight. I asked my family doctor about the twenty extra pounds I was carrying. He asked me what I ate and was skeptical when I pulled out a food diary with entries such as this:

Breakfast:

Bagel, toasted, dry

Orange juice

Iced tea

Lunch:

Turkey breast on whole-wheat bun, fat-free mayonnaise, tomato and lettuce.

Apple

Skimmed milk

Dinner

Pasta with Marinara sauce

Salad greens with lemon juice

Bread, dry

Skimmed milk.

Snacks:

Fat-free muffin

Fat-free yogurt

Orange

The doctor sighed, asked if I was picking food off my daughters' plates, binge-eating at night or maybe just sitting around too much.

Within six months, I had outgrown my size twelve jeans. Still haunted by the memory of those size fourteen pink pants, I refused to buy jeans in a larger size and started wearing sweat pants instead.

Again I asked my doctor: why? He tested me for diabetes, low thyroid and, since he was running the tests anyway, re-checked my cholesterol.

My blood sugar and thyroid were fine. My cholesterol was up 20 points – still in the low normal range – but how could that be? When I was eating eggs, red meat and butter every day, my count was below normal. Now I was following a fat-free vegan diet, and my cholesterol level had increased? Why, doctor, why?

He shrugged, asked again if I was hiding anything from him. He said maybe my heredity was catching up with me – my father weighed nearly 300 pounds – and I'd just have to try harder to lose weight.

I read and read and read some more about diet and health, and everything and everyone preached the benefits of carbohydrates and the evils of fat. I was constantly hungry, chronically fatigued – and getting fatter by the month.

My only consolation is that I was healthy and my daughters would be healthy, too. Their diet wasn't as austere as mine – I'd also read the literature that said kids need fat and protein – but peanut butter and yogurt took care of those requirements. Maybe I was a little fat, but I was a good mom.

Two years later, I was a lot fat – I weighed 180 – and doubted my parenting skills. My daughters were gaining weight too.

By this time I'd moved from the Midwest to Manhattan. I walked five miles a day and passed up nearly every culinary experience the city had to offer. My unexciting diet consisted of a bagel in the morning, an appetizer portion of steamed vegetable dumplings in the afternoon, and a veggie burger or pasta in the evening.

I stopped gaining weight, but I didn't lose an ounce.

Went to another doctor, who asked the same questions, reacted with the same skepticism to my answers ("C'mon, what are you eating after everyone's asleep at night?")

I was a big, fat, unhealthy failure. The only thing getting smaller was my self-esteem. But what I couldn't resolve was why I was eating so little and weighing so much – and feeling doubted rather than helped by those in the healing profession.

I offered them theories – perhaps years of stress had wreaked havoc on my metabolism or perhaps I was eating too little and my metabolism had slowed to "starvation mode" – and their reactions ranged from derision to polite interest.

I gave up. I resigned myself to a life of obesity. Tired of being hungry, I started eating more. More rice, more pasta, more bread. I baked cookies and cake and pie. And it didn't seem to make much difference. My weight was high – way too high – but it was steady and at least I wasn't feeling so food-deprived.

I moved from the East coast to the West, began working from home, and stopped looking in the mirror. I walked two to three miles a day, worked out with weights three times a week, and consoled myself with the fact that my eating habits were earth and animal friendly. And healthy! The American Heart Association and medical wisdom told me so. Every doctor, nurse and dietitian I met approved my diet – they just didn't believe I followed it.

Six months ago, Sandy approached me with her idea for a book, told me the story about losing – and keeping off – forty pounds by giving up all the things I was eating. Then she sent me two books, the Schwarzbein Principle and Dr. Atkin's Diet Revolution.

I read both, started thinking about my own diet history – thin when I ate a lot of protein, fat when I ate a lot of carbohydrates – and felt angry, confused -- and hopeful.

Angry that my rigid adherence to the medically sanctioned diet may have been responsible for an unhealthy weight gain, confused that such a universally accepted theory could be so wrong and hopeful that I could give up my plus-size figure for the one I wanted – and deserved!

Two weeks later, I ate a piece of meat, my first in ten years. It was a tough, painful decision. I'd become a committed vegetarian during the past decade. Although my motivation had been better health, I saw the humane value in my food choices and couldn't easily abandon them.

I know that there are non-meat protein options for vegetarians, but I am allergic to soy, dairy and most nuts. I get nauseated if I eat more than a half an egg at a time. So I added a little meat (about two to three ounces of chicken or turkey a day), forced myself to eat a half an egg twice a day, and stopped eating bread (but kept rice and pasta in my diet.)

I've lost thirty pounds!

My younger daughter bought me a pair of size twelve jeans for Christmas – the first jeans I've owned in five years – and they're loose!

After ten years of gains, I'm finally losing.

By ignoring what I'd been taught and paying attention to what actually works.

My "diet" isn't the same as the one described by Sandy or prescribed by my doctors. And I still don't know what foods I will end up eating on a consistent basis; I have not refined or fully tested my own diet theory.

The point is that the diet I choose will be my own, the one that works best for me. Sandy's phone call inspired me to become my own weight-loss guru rather than become a disciple of any single diet prophet. She showed me how to live against the grain (whether literally or figuratively) and become the master of my own diet destiny.

Chapter Four:
We Get it, Now Let's Get Going!

OK, now that you've been introduced to Ellen and me, it's time to learn more about the most important person in your exciting new journey toward permanent weight loss: you!

This is the part of the book that starts to get a little bit hard, the part that may make you uncomfortable and consequently lead you to glaze over and lose interest. It may tap into that self-loathing fat person mentality that elastic waistbands and avoidance of full-length mirrors can't hide. This is when you have to come to grips with the fact that this book is really about you.

You're inspired, I hope, by my weight-management success and how I conquered my weight-loss struggle by giving up grains, and how Ellen is discovering the joy (and pound-reduction) of a simplified, sane approach to eating. Before you can begin your path, you need to honestly answer some questions about your past and current eating habits. Maybe you know where you want to end up on your weight-loss travels, but you can't get there from here until you know where *here* is. You can't map out your dietary goals without identifying a starting point.

To find out where you are, ask yourself the following questions:

1. Do I eat too much?

If you're overweight, the answer seems obvious, of course! How did I become a size fourteen unless I stuffed my face with fat-inducing poison (AKA, Hershey's kisses, Sara Lee cheesecake, etc.) because skinny people never overeat?

Stop right there! Maybe you DO overeat (and you're about to find out) and maybe (more likely) you are eating the wrong foods; However, it's also possible you eat too little. If you've ever been on a starvation diet, your body kicks into survival mode by slowing down your metabolism and hanging onto all the fat it can. That's why you can always lose weight on fad diets – and always end up gaining back more than you lost: your body, when it finally gets a morsel of real nutrition, stores it away for the next time you get hooked on a diet-of-the month. If you've been doing this for many years, your body may be conditioned to store extra fat in anticipation of your next famine. You may discover that you need to eat more **of the right foods** in order to lose weight successfully.

But how much is too much?

What works for your best friend may not work for you. Our metabolisms are not created equally. It's not fair, certainly, but get over it! We all know super-skinny people who can eat anything and everything without gaining an ounce. You already know that you can't. Don't blame yourself – you're not a bad person because you weigh thirty pounds more than the ideal – and don't blame fate either – your heredity plays a role in how likely you are to be thin or heavy, but unlike the color of your eyes, your weight is a genetic trait you can do something about.

So, don't hate your thin friends and don't judge yourself by their standards. You're just different.

Each of us gets handed a different set of fat or skinny genes. It's then up to us what we do with them. It will only drive you crazy to compare your eating habits with someone whose genetic history is totally different than yours. So you either have to give up the comparison or give up skinny friends.

And since you're on your way to becoming one of those lean ladies, it's better to change your attitude than your companions!

But it's essential that you 'fess' up to how much you eat and what you're eating. So keep track!

If you've ever kept a food journal before and found it tiresome and guilt-inducing, you're not alone. But try to think of this exercise as a snapshot of what IS, not a judgment about you, your eating habits, your willpower or anything else. Call it a food record. Record implies simplicity. And keep in mind: when I say food record, I don't care if you write it on paper, type in on your keyboard, imprint it on your brain or stitch it on a pillowcase! It doesn't matter HOW you keep your record. The idea is to start thinking about what you eat and being accountable for it.

And you don't have to keep a food record forever. If you eat the same things day after day, you can probably keep a three-day record of what you are eating and call it quits. If you eat radically different on weekends, be sure to include Saturday and Sunday to get an accurate assessment. If your eating patterns vary a lot – depending on your menstrual cycle, your boss's mood, the status of your love life, the amount of freeway traffic, your luck playing the lottery or whether your favorite show was interrupted by a news bulletin – you might want to keep a longer-term food record.

For however long you record your eating pattern, though, be vigilant. If you eat a 14-ounce bag of chips and the serving size is 1 ounce, be honest! Count it as fourteen servings and not two or three. You're the only one who's going to read it, so don't try to fool yourself.

Once you've completed the food record, use the calorie/ carbohydrate counter on the following pages to add up your day-to-day intake of carbohydrates and calories. When I did this, it proved a revelation. The foods that I couldn't control, the foods that were most often high in carbohydrates and calories, all contained flour! For me, eliminating flour meant eliminating the problems that I believe make me fat - high calorie and high carbohydrate foods. The purpose of this is not to turn you into a food math expert – but to give you an honest view of your current eating habits and a clearer understanding of how changing your eating habits will help you achieve permanent weight loss.

If your caloric intake is reasonable but your carb intake is high, for instance, it will help you appreciate the importance of changing *what* you eat, rather than *how much* you eat. The chart provides information for about 1000 foods so, if you don't find precisely what you're looking for (if you eat a different brand of cereal) you should find a close-enough match for the purposes of doing your pre-slim homework.

And, for those of you who do eat the whole pie, the entire cake, the full quart of ice cream, we've made the math simple for you. Our calorie/gram counter will tell you, for instance, that there are 2285 calories and 330 grams of carbohydrates in a blueberry pie as well as 380 calories and 55 grams in a single slice.

Once you complete the food record, you should also be able to answer the next question:

2. Are there trigger foods that set off bad eating patterns for me?

When you review your food record, did you find that you were doing fine until, say Day 5, when you accepted a coworker's offer of a teeny, tiny bite-sized brownie that was part of a platter of goodies set out during a morning conference? Did one bite lead to two? Did two bites lead to six (which was really just one brownie, the pieces were so tiny) which made it OK to finish every last piece on the plate? Did your chocolate craving continue so that you had to go home and bake yourself a batch of brownies (and eat them before anyone discovered your guilty secret)? Or did you try to stop the craving by eating everything BUT chocolate? Maybe a bag of corn chips, a box of doughnuts, a plate of lasagna…?

If certain foods trigger overeating, stop eating those foods. Now. Forever. You just can't have them!

Again, I speak from experience.

About six months elapsed between the writing of the first chapter and this one. Remember I told you that I hadn't touched flour in seven years and had kept my size six figure for all that time? All true.

Then, during the recent holidays, I let a few chips slip into my diet. After seven years, what harm could a few chips do, right? I wasn't going to blow everything I'd worked for because of 50 to 100 calories' worth of deep-fried potatoes.

Except, that single handful of chips brought back the old cravings. I tried a couple bites of chocolate –just a couple – but as I popped that first kiss into my mouth part of me knew it wouldn't stop at one or two, and it didn't. Before long, my cravings had flared up.

As the desire for crunchy and starchy foods started building, I began overeating everything. I thought I could keep away from the forbidden foods by binging on those that were allowed. But I wanted all of those foods – and the demon foods, too!

It wasn't long before my favorite pair of jeans didn't button so easily, before I decided I didn't really want to wear those jeans anyway and a looser-fitting pair of pants suddenly became my choice.

And, then I told myself, that for me, there is no "little of this" or "tiny bit of that" when it comes to my trigger foods. And if you have trigger foods, the same wisdom applies to you. Identify the triggers – and say goodbye to them.

You eat a little and you eventually want more and more. Then you end up eating bigger portions of everything just to tame that beast! Of course this leads to weight gain and the old cycle begins. In my case, I (temporarily) lost a sense of that body, mind, spirit connection that kept me grounded to the no-flour commitment.

When I lost that connection, I gained weight – and guilt. Boy did that suck! But I didn't look for a quick fix and I didn't give in to defeat. I returned to the eating habits that kept me lean for seven years – the eating habits I will share with you – and guess what? It worked. I went back to the basic guiding principle that I adopted seven years ago: STAY AWAY! Foods that contain flour, bad fats

& gobs of sugar simply don't exist in my world. I'm much happier without them. Period.

For us lifelong overeaters, it is simpler, easier and more effective to just stay away from trigger foods than to try to control how we eat these foods. When I put back even a small portion of these nasty "fake" foods, inevitably they drive my eating. When I take them away completely, I choose my eating, and that makes me a happy lean person.

If you've identified trigger foods while compiling your food record, you've identified a behavior problem. You have to change the behavior in order to permanently change your weight. If you've been trigger-hungry more than once in the past (and for most of us, the habit repeats itself with devastating frequency) accept this about yourself.

Then answer the final question of this chapter?

3. Do I want to choose what I eat or do I want food to control me?

Don't be a food victim. Don't let homemade biscuits, store-bought cupcakes (or whatever your trigger-food may be) determine how you eat, how you look or how you feel about yourself. Choose your eating. Choose to be happy, healthy and slim, not for a week or a month, but from this moment forward.

Be honest with – and kind to – yourself. Use your food record as a research tool. In the next several chapters, we share some popular dieting theories. See how your habits fit (or don't fit) the experts' advice. Did you eat a ton of carbs and practically no fat (the way the experts told you to eat for the past two decades)? Did you find yourself still fat after giving up egg yolks, red meat, butter, cheese and every oil except olive? Have you tried Atkins and had a quick weight loss? Did you maintain that loss? Or did you give up because you started craving the good carbohydrates like fruit and vegetables -- how can a carrot be bad for you? Or maybe you are afraid to try Atkins – wasn't he the heart attack doctor? – and are you confused about why this once-maligned doctor is so popular again?

When you find your own body, mind, spirit connection, you will find out the truth behind the diet fallacy and why you haven't failed these diets: the diets have failed you..

End the failure. Design a diet that fits you – and keeps you fit.

You will find a carb/calorie counter in the back of the book. Please use it as a reference ONLY to complete your food record and help you change your eating patterns. But don't think you have to use it daily. What I'm showing you is a permanent lifestyle change, and you can't get that from a piece of paper.

Part Two:

De-tangling the Diet Triangle

The Loaf: Love, Leave or Leaf it?
Three Leading Weight Loss Theories

Chapter Five:
The Protein Machine

When Dr. Robert Atkins introduced his protein-rich, carbohydrate-poor diet thirty years ago, he was criticized by calorie-counting doctors and adored by millions of desperatos who couldn't lose weight no matter how well they kept to their carrot-stick-and-cottage-cheese diets. Dr. Atkins told overweight, guilt-laden Americans what no one had ever told them before: you're not eating too much, you're just eating the wrong foods! He told them to eat more – as much as they wanted – of meat, cheese, butter and cream – and to enjoy a cocktail or two as well.

It seemed too good to be true (but that never stopped a dieter before) but what surprised everyone – including Dr. Atkins's many detractors – is that it worked. People lost weight and, if they stuck with Atkins, kept it off.

As Ellen remembers:

"My father had lost and regained 80 pounds several times over by the time I was a young teen, and I was dreading his latest no-carb kick. How could a diet that told him it was OK to have steak and martinis possibly work? Or that he could drench his salads in blue cheese dressing or slather whipped cream over strawberries? But he did lose weight and kept it off for eight years. And then his doctor told him to eliminate red meat and add fiber to his diet."

Dr. Atkins earned fame and grudging respect during the 1970s, even though the medical community didn't quite understand HOW his diet worked and many suspected the Atkins diet was really a low-calorie diet in disguise (because appetite suppression occurs naturally with a protein-dense diet). Many owed their svelte frames to the doctor who prescribed an all-you-can-eat approach to everything except carbohydrates – grains, fruit, sugar – which were severely restricted. In Dr. Atkins's world, fat was good; flour and sugar were bad.

Ten years later, doctors introduced their patients to a new health concern – cholesterol – and when blood tests showed scary levels of fat clogging people's arteries, the American diet was to blame.

Fat makes us fat, we were told, and animal fat makes us fat in the worst way – sends those triglyceride counts to heart-attack levels. Dr. Atkins and red meat were out, oat bran and pasta were in.

Overnight, dieters were told to flip their eating habits, to eat lots of bread (but without butter) and tons of pasta (with olive oil or marinara sauce, but no meat). It was impossible to reconcile an Atkins or other high-protein diet with the new medical wisdom, so people threw away their carbohydrate gram counters, started reading fat content labels, and reaching for rice cakes instead of cheese slices between meals.

A funny (not-so-funny) thing happened. A lot of people started to gain weight on the heart-healthy diets their doctors prescribed. Eat better carbs -- whole grains instead of white flour – and exercise more. So people did that, but, twenty bowls of brown rice and dozens of 2-for-1 gym memberships later, many of these people were still porky even if they hadn't eaten an ounce of pig's meat in years.

Today, Dr. Atkins has revolutionized our thinking once again, and advertisers can't tell you often or loudly enough that *their* products are Atkins approved low-carb. But his popularity is not without controversy. A medical examiner's report into the death of the doctor – he died in April, 2003, after slipping on an icy patch of sidewalk – indicated he had a history of heart attack, heart failure and hypertension.

According to the report released to the Wall Street Journal by a pro-vegetarian group, he was also more than fifty pounds overweight.

But the Atkins camp counters this with evidence that the doctor's heart problems were connected to a virus, that he had no record of a heart attack and that much of his weight gain was due to fluid retention, common to someone with a weak heart.

So, what is the Atkins diet that has created so much hype and criticism and why is it supposed to work?

The Atkins diet, if adopted for life as the doctor recommends, is actually four diets: The Induction, Ongoing Weight Loss, Pre-Maintenance and Maintenance. Many dieters -- and most of Atkins's detractors -- consider only the first phase -- the eat-a-ton-of-bacon segment -- and ignore the rest.

The Induction is a 14-day diet that bans nearly all carbohydrates (it's pretty much meat and salad) and puts the body into a state of ketosis, which forces the body to burn fat. This metabolic advantage is the key to a rapid weight reduction Atkins' followers expect to enjoy in their first two weeks. Two pleasant side effects - reduced hunger and increased energy. People who adhere to Atkins (and true devotees carry urine dipsticks in their pockets to measure their ketosis levels on a regular basis) for fourteen days are expected to be so delighted with the results that they fall easily into the second phase.

During the Ongoing Weight Loss phase, dieters can slightly increase their consumption of carbohydrates. The amount of recommended carbs varies depending on a person's metabolic resistance but may include up to 40 grams of carbohydrates a day. (Metabolic resistance is why some people find it harder to lose weight than others. The rate of weight loss should be less than in the Induction phase, but still consistent. If a person stops losing – or starts gaining – it's time to cut back on the carbohydrates.

The next phase is Pre-Maintenance. This is a transition period between reaching your target weight and adopting a lifetime stay-slim plan. A person in this phase slowly adds carbohydrates to the diet. Maybe a person was losing weight on 35 carbs a day and will be able to maintain that weight at 60 carbs a day. But adding 25 carbs to a diet is extreme and may lead to weight gain. For one thing, with the extra carbs comes increased appetite (you're no longer in ketosis) and there's a danger of triggering old overeating as you seek to satisfy new hunger pangs. By gradually increasing carbs, your body – and appetite – can adjust to the new way of eating.

The final Maintenance phase is your for-life diet and may include bread and potatoes daily for some; others may find they have to limit such food to a few times a week. If you look at the calorie/carb counter in the last chapter you can see the marked difference between a 20-grams-a-day Induction diet and a 60-grams-a-day Maintenance plan.

Atkins cites six reasons for his diet's success:

1. Creates fat mobilization. A body in ketosis burns fat, and a diet that contains almost exclusively protein and fat, creates ketosis. Carbohydrates, on the other hand, produce insulin, which makes fat.

2. The diet satisfies hunger. There is never a reason to starve, because you can eat as much fish, chicken, meat, eggs and most cheese as you want.

3. The metabolic defect involving insulin can be circumvented by restricting carbohydrates, avoiding the problem that makes people fat.

4. The correction to metabolism is so great that people can lose weight while consuming higher calories than in carbohydrate-heavy diets.

5. Diets high in carbohydrates are what most dieters don't need and can't become slim on. People whose metabolisms are resistant to weight loss are likely people who create too much insulin when they consume carbohydrates. And someone who has food triggers or carb cravings likely has this resistance.

6. A carbohydrate-restricted diet dissolves fat, making it even more effective (and much more pleasant) than fasting.

Dr. Atkins's message: "If you're overweight, you're not greedy, not weak-willed, not lazy, not self-indulgent, not awful but in all probability, metabolically unfortunate" should make him every dieter's hero, even if you don't accept the rest of his weight-reduction theory.

Personally, I think Dr. Atkins is more right than wrong, and I applaud his recent vindication (as evidenced by the growing amount of grocery-shelf space allocated to Atkins's fare); However, I find fault with him on two counts:

First, he acknowledges that many fat people are addicted to carbohydrates – particularly refined carbs such as those found in cakes, cookies, breads and pasta – and that consuming these foods creates both metabolic resistance and overeating. Why, then, does he allow any to creep back into people's diets? I know (as I shared in the previous chapter) that there is no such thing as "a little" of my forbidden foods. I am addicted to flour products and must STAY AWAY from all of them all of the time, forever. When I did try Atkins and stuck with it to the letter, it worked. The "sticking to it part" was the problem. Dr. Atkins didn't take into account my emotional and intellectual lifestyle, and this is why I believe that Atkins' inclusion of grain products is a flaw in an otherwise credible low-carbohydrate theory.

I also think Atkins went too far in promoting a high-fat diet. I KNOW my lifestyle does not support unlimited consumption of red meat and whipped cream. Although he backs away somewhat from his "fat is good" theory in his latest book, Atkins still recommends cholesterol-laden foods in amounts higher than make me comfortable. Although my "no more flour" credo is compatible with and simpler than Atkin's carbohydrate-counting system, I believe in being sensible about cholesterol. I include more chicken than steak in my diet, and am careful about things such as cheese and butter. Atkins would get stronger support from me – and less skepticism from a press that leaks medical reports – if he'd taken a softer stance about the fat issue. The way I see it, a calorie is a calorie. If you don't burn it, you store it. Period.

Recent research is validating his research about carbs, and maybe he'll yet be proven right about butter and fois gras as well, but until I'm convinced that eating more fat is actually good for me, I'll put more faith in Pam than pate.

I also believe it's critical to choose the *right* carbohydrates if you want to maintain your weight, a distinction Atkins ignores. For example, an apple -- a big, beautiful Granny Smith apple is better than a slice of French bread. The French bread actually has slightly fewer carbs than the apple, BUT it has more calories AND you are likely to eat more bread than fruit (wouldn't you be mad if the server at your favorite restaurant gave you a single-slice bread basket?) And that's why I don't eat flour, rice and starchy fruits and vegetables such as avocados, bananas and corn. And that's why I don't think you should either.

Chapter Six:
Bran Fans

The most popular, widely touted health theory of the twentieth century – the low-fat, high-carbohydrate diet -- was, until recently, accepted as fact by most of the medical community. Introduced in the 1980s and embraced by our family doctors who, until then, were mostly ignorant about nutrition, this theory promised that we could be healthy and thin without ever going hungry.

It was the promise of health – at a time when cholesterol counts had reached cocktail party-level awareness – that turned us away from red meat and into fans of all things bran. The idea that fat makes people fat made simple sense. It didn't take much imagination to picture how the marbled fat in a filet mignon could clog our arteries.

So, it was out with protein and in with carbs. Although hard to accept at first – America was a nation of meat-eaters, after all – most of us made the switch. We started eating more (skinless) chicken and fish and we were encouraged to give up animal products entirely, replacing them with pasta and rice or, if you really needed a protein fix, soy.

As hard as it was to give up bacon and eggs, the comfort of carbs was appealing. We could eat more bread, just without butter. But let's face it, rolls hot from the oven tasted pretty good – and even better with fat-free preserves) and once-scorned sugar was suddenly our friend. Want to eat a pound of licorice? Go ahead, its fat-free! An entire Entenmann's fat-free coffee cake? Yes, we don't count calories any more. Just fat. We could eat much more of anything and everything as long as we kept our fat intake to a minimum.

Why didn't this work? Why didn't we, as a nation of carbophiles, live longer, healthier and skinnier lives?

Several reasons:

First, to be fair to the pro-carbohydrate medical community, no one ever advocated an all-you-can-eat pancake (and syrup!) diet. The food regimen that was supposed to work was one that included whole and complex carbohydrates such as green vegetables, brown rice and kidney beans. These are slower to digest (and thus more satisfying) than refined (white flour and sugar) carbohydrates and less likely to produce food cravings. Also, the high-fiber content in these foods were designed to cleanse our systems and reduce toxicity.

There are some people – vegetarians mostly – for whom the high-carbohydrate diet did what it was supposed to do, reduced cholesterol and weight. But most of us did not trade in our burgers for bulgar wheat, most of us did not sign on for a steady diet of steamed kale.

And Madison Avenue told us we didn't have to. The power of marketing is the second key reason why the low-fat diet failed us.

Carboyhdrates don't count, only fat the advertisers claimed. Eat plenty of pasta, keep the (air-popped) popcorn coming, and keep your candy bowl full. (Remember all those fat-free labels on Skittles and Lifesavers?) Just stay away from fat, and you'll be healthy and lean.

The problem with this theory is that all carbohydrates are sugar. Cake and other simple carbohydrates break down more quickly than complex ones such as those found in fruits, but they all end up as sugar in the body. Our bodies metabolize sugar quickly, and just as swiftly turn the excess sugar into fat.

How does this work?

Dr. Diana Schwarzbein, whose research into metabolism stemmed from concerns that diabetics were getting sicker on the low-fat, high-carbohydrate diets recommended by their physicians, explains that the way our body uses carbohydrates is determined by the ratio of insulin to glucagons produced in our pancreas.

Glucagon mobilizes nutrients, directing the liver to release sugar, which raises the levels of blood sugar available for the brain and body. Glucagon also directs cells to release fat that can be used as energy and to release proteins that can be used as building materials.

Insulin is responsible for nutrient storage. Insulin puts nutrients into cells, refueling the body and balancing blood-sugar levels, which protects the brain. Insulin also tells the liver that too much sugar has entered and the liver reacts by increasing fat production from the incoming sugar.

The ratio between these two hormones determines whether food will be used as building materials, fuel or stored as fat, Dr. Schwarzbein writes in the *Schwarzbein Principle*. A low ratio (a higher percentage of glucagons, which is released in response to protein) means that more food will be used as building material or fuel. A high ratio (a high ratio of insulin, which is released in response to sugar) means that more food will be stored as fat.

So, even though a piece of chicken or a cookie may contain the same amount of calories when sitting on the counter, our bodies use those calories in different ways. Most of the calories in chicken will be used to build tissue, but the calories in the cookie are destined to turn into fat.

The other problem with the high-carbohydrate diet is that, because it is digested so easily, we get hungry more often (kicking in the carb cravings that cause so many of us trouble). What's even worse, Dr. Schwarzbein says, is that our bodies protect us from eating too much protein and fat but don't prevent us from binging on carbohydrates. This means that it's really difficult to finish eating a steak when you're full, but all too simple to polish off a bag of donuts even when we're not hungry.

Carbohydrates do not stay in the stomach. They go right through your stomach and into the small intestine. You do not experience stomach distention or the release of cholecystokinin (a hormone that tells your brain that food is coming and makes your gallbladder contract, secreting bile to help absorb fats). Carbohydrates must enter the bloodstream before triggering the release of insulin, which causes a temporary release of serotonin in the brain, signaling the beginning of satiety. Next, the sugar leaves the liver and goes to the brain. At that point, your brain-sugar level rises, signaling that you are fully satiated. But carbohydrates have to go through the entire digestive and absorptive process before the brain understands it is getting food and stops sending hunger signals, and by that time you could have eaten an entire box of cereal. Whereas eating protein and fats signals the brain early on to stop demanding food, with carbohydrates there is no early regulation to say, 'Don't eat any more.'

So, if carbohydrates cause so many people to overeat, how did the high-carb diet stay in favor so long?

First, a high-carb diet, like almost any diet, works in the beginning. When we overload on sugar, our body draws on its muscle glycogen stores, and the first few pounds fall right off. This early weight loss coupled with the feel-good serotonin levels supplied by carbohydrates encouraged many people to continue. And for awhile, the weight loss continued as well, but much of the weight lost was lean body mass, not fat.

Eventually, for most people, the weight loss ended and many found themselves getting more body fat around the middle (the midsection is the body's insulin meter, and prolonged consumption of high carbohydrates produces high insulin levels.) What to do? Family doctors told us to exercise more (which probably eliminated more muscle, not fat). Then, even worse, our bodies, in an attempt to slow down the self-destruction, slowed down our metabolism. Depending on our base metabolic structure, we ended up too thin with a high body-fat composition or too fat with a high body-fat composition. Some of us looked better than others on a high-carbohydrate diet, but all of us were too fat, Dr. Schwarzbein says.

If you're reading this book, you know the low-fat, high-carbohydrate diet didn't make you slimmer – and may have made you heavier. What you may not have known – until now – is that none of the weight gain was your fault. Carbohydrates are designed to produce fat, and unless you have a fat-resistant metabolism, that's exactly what they did to you and me. The carbohydrates were just doing their job – and we've got the hips to prove it!

Fortunately, I found a solution– no more flour – and in the next section, I'll show you just how satisfying and simple this solution can be for you. But first, I want to introduce you to one more popular dieting theory (though if you like food as much as I do, you may find it hard to imagine, much less digest).

Chapter Seven:
The Raw Truth

As Kermit the Frog can attest, "Its not easy being green." And outside of celebrity and vegetarian circles, the garden-rich component of the raw diet may seem more radical (or ridiculous) than about radicchio. It may take a personal chef and/or a great deal of devotion to spend a lifetime on this diet. What works for Demi Moore, Woody Harrelson, Alicia Silverstone and Sting, for instance, may not work for those of us who don't have a cook to ensure that the broccoli we eat is never heated beyond a temperature of 118 degrees. And a personal trainer to keep us away from other, more palatable food choices. The raw diet definitely stems from an eat-to-live philosophy, and you probably won't find too much that you can eat at many restaurants. But it does have a lot of healthy attributes, so pour yourself a shot of wheat grass and get ready to Go Green!

Green Is In!

Apart from St. Patrick's Day or a Dr. Seuss theme party, when's the last time you ate something green for breakfast? If you're like most people, it's probably been a long time – maybe forever – since you began your day eating a bowl of broccoli or a plate of spinach (minus the eggs and cheese in an omelet).

In a raw diet, green goes with everything at every meal. The goal of the diet is to maintain alkalinity in your body. If you want to try any or all of the teachings of the raw advocates, make the transition a slow one. No one, including the authors quoted in this chapter, made the transition from carnivore to herbivore overnight, and some continue to include red (and other) meats in their diet.

Your goal is to reduce acid and increase alkaline in your body. This chapter tells you why and how to strive to achieve the ideal balance.

The Magic pH for Maximum Energy

Some followers believe that breakthrough research by Dr. Robert Young has given us some guidelines as to ideal alkalinity. Most of us have highly acidic blood. When our bodies have a pH balance of 7.35, it operates at peak efficiency. When our bodies are more acidic, we compensate in an effort to restore the balance. The effort robs us of energy as the acid does what acid does – it destroys. Hydrochloric acid can burn a hole through marble. Just imagine what it can do to your blood vessels!

Alkaline lines the blood vessel walls with a protective fat coating to neutralize acid. The goal of "good" cholesterol is just that, to protect us from acid.

When we put too much acid in our system, however, we overtax our natural protection.

What kinds of foods create acid and which promote alkalinity? The chart on the next page gives you specifics, but here are some basics:

Meats, pasta, breads and dairy all are considered acidic. Surprised? Something such as bread seems an unlikely culprit in acid production – most breads *taste* sweet – but it's what happens to a food once it's digested that puts it in the category of acid or alkaline.

Green foods promote alkalinity. When our bodies are properly pH balanced, we aren't working so hard to regain the balance and, thus, have a LOT of energy in reserve for joyful living rather than blood cleansing.

How do you tell when you've reached the magic 7.35? A blood test is the most accurate method, but a more convenient method is to take a urine sample. (anyone who's ever tried Dr. Atkins's diet may already have a supply of "dip sticks" used to detect ketosis, but you can get the sticks and the litmus paper to test for acid/alkaline from your pharmacist). You can also test your saliva.

If your pre-meal saliva pH is between 6.8 and 5.5, you're in a favorable to acceptable Ph-zone.

If your saliva pH is 5.5-5.8 before a meal and stays the same after a meal, your body is extremely acidic and you are without adequate reserves. At this point, for instance, it could be dangerous to exercise strenuously. Your body simply cannot handle the stress.

If your saliva pH goes down after a meal, it has been affected by emotions that are distorting your physiology. If you remain stuck in this mode – anger, frustration, fear or other negative attitudes –those acid thoughts can lead to disease.

If you're still with me -- and this is the simplified version! -- you are better at saliva-testing than I could ever be.

Green Goes with Everything

It is important to remember to make your dietary adjustments gradually. One way to do this is to put more balance in each of your meals. Rather than have meat and potatoes for instance (both acidic), have meat and a salad or potatoes and Brussels sprouts. Limit your acidic foods to one item per meal. And if you're ever in doubt as to what to mix with what, remember that green goes with everything! Think rice and (green) beans, bread with avocado, chicken with peas. It is a French culinary tradition that every plate should include something green. Whether they were considering the aesthetics or the alkalinity, it's a good rule to remember. At every meal, put something green on your plate. (and eat it!)

What's acidic and what's not? See the chart on the next pages. It's not whether a food begins as an acid; it's how it ends up in your system that's important. Lemons, for instance, are definitely acidic when you bite into them, but they produce an alkaline ash in your body.

Foods that Promote Alkalinity

(Foods that are good!)

Almonds	Dates, dried
Apples	Figs, dried
Apricots	Grapefruit
Avocados	Grapes
Bananas	Green beans
Beans, dried	Green peas
Beet greens	Lemons
Beets	Lettuce
Blackberries	Lima beans, dried
Broccoli	Lima beans, green
Brussels sprouts	Limes
Cabbage	Milk, goat*
Carrots	Millet
Cauliflower	Molasses
Celery	Mushrooms
Chard leaves	Muskmelon
Cherries, sour	Onions
Cucumbers	Oranges

Parsnips	Rutabaga
Peaches	Sauerkraut
Pears	Soybeans, green
Pineapple	Spinach, raw
Potatoes, sweet	Strawberries
Potatoes, white	Tangerines
Radishes	Tomatoes
Raisins	Watercress
Raspberries	Watermelon

Neutral ash foods
(that have an acidifying effect)

Corn oil

Corn syrup

Refined sugar

Olive Oil

(What's the difference between a neutral and an acid ash food? I don't know! They all end up the same in your body! But the petri-dish inspired proponents of the raw diet insist on making the distinction. Me, I'd rather concentrate on the spice, aroma and flavor of my food, but here's the info anyway-- enjoy!)

Acid Ash Foods

(Foods to Avoid/Limit)

Bacon	Milk, cow *
Barley	Macaroni
Beef	Oatmeal
Blueberries	Oysters
Bran, wheat	Peanut Butter
Bran, oat	Peanuts
Bread, white,	Peas, dried
Bread, whole wheat	Pike
Butter	Plums*
Carob	Pork
Cheese	Prunes*
Chicken	Rice, brown
Codfish	Rice, white
Corn	Salmon
Corned beef	Sardines
Crackers, soda	Sausage
Cranberries *	Scallops
Currants	Shrimp
Eggs	Spaghetti
Flour, white	Squash, winter
Flour, whole wheat	Sunflower seeds
Haddock	Turkey
Honey	Veal
Lamb	Walnuts
Lentils, dried	Wheat germ
Lobster	Yogurt

Raw Foods for Raw Energy

As you gradually progress into an alkaline diet, you are supposed to realize several motivating benefits:

If you are overweight, proponents of the raw diet say, you will lose weight without hunger. When our bodies remain properly balanced, our appetite decreases. When our bodies are acidic, our bodies are looking for a way to compensate and we crave more energy. We may be tempted to fill those cravings with junk food and caffeinated beverages. Eliminate the imbalance and you eliminate the cravings. You will no longer feel deprived of sweets and sodas – you will have tons of energy without them.

You will feel better! Traditional dieting often makes us look fit but feel lousy. When we boost our alkaline levels, we boost our health. If eating raw almonds and carrots for lunch makes us feel nourished rather than deprived, we'll start to look forward to our alkaline-rich meals.

This progression should also lead you to eat more raw and fewer cooked foods. If this seems beyond comprehension today, that's OK. Soup for breakfast – lukewarm soup no less – is a far cry from the Egg McMuffin you may be accustomed to eating. Your body has adapted to this bad diet, and it has to be retrained.

John Robbins, author of *Diet for a New World*, is, for instance, a strong advocate of eating habits that are healthy both for you and the environment, but he doesn't suggest you go from meat three times a week to tofu twice a day.

Robbins lists 124 -- yes 124!! -- action steps you can take to begin the path toward wellness. I couldn't imagine implementing more than two of them (sponsoring an alkaline-rich picnic -- come on!). But in the interest of being as informational as I promised, here are twelve to give you an idea:

1. Set a good example for your children (and this will be good for you too!) by preparing more meals from the four "new world" food groups – grains, legumes, fruits and vegetables.
2. Replace the junk food in your pantry with healthy snacks in your refrigerator.
3. Buy produce from farmers markets and local produce stands. Even if the food isn't organically grown, it is less likely to have been heavily treated with chemicals because it didn't have to travel far from field to market.
4. You can ask your favorite restaurants to prepare meat-free dishes and thank them (by returning often and telling others) when they do.
5. Eat more dark green and yellow vegetables, which contain cancer-fighting agents such as betacaratene.
6. Try substituting rice milk, soy milk or almond milk for cow's milk. Begin by including it in recipes and work

your way up to adding it to cereal and eventually drinking it as a beverage. All are rich in calcium and protein.

7. Save the cooking water from cooking vegetables. Use it as a base for soups and sauces.

8. Ask your grocer about the chemicals used on fresh produce. The more you ask, the more likely you are to bring about positive change.

9. Introduce friends and family to your newfound ideas by sharing your lunch or sponsoring a picnic.

10. Start paying attention to what other people are saying about food. Point out the myths when you recognize them. By educating others, you will learn more yourself.

11. Order vegetarian meals when traveling on airplanes. And keep asking for the specific foods you'd like to see offered. Ask for alkaline-rich foods often enough, and someone will pay attention (says the author!).

12. Celebrate your healthier eating habits by serving meals with an eye for aesthetics and ambiance. Candlelight and an attractive table make an important difference in your enjoyment.

Chewing the Fat

Green is great, but don't forget the fat. Fat is not the enemy in a raw diet! Fatty acids have the power to relieve pain. We need them.

Yes, we need fats for brain function, but fats also literally reduce inflammation, allow the transfer of oxygen and - super bonus – boost our energy!

Fish, almonds and avocados are good sources of essential fatty acids. If you don't like eating any of these, you can take fish oil capsules. Essential fatty acids won't make you fat, they will make you healthy.

What happens to our body when we do not have enough fat? Experts tell us we become vulnerable to high blood pressure and high triglycerides; we have difficulty learning and suffer from poor motor skills and behavioral changes. Our immune system falters, our skin dries and we sweat excessively. We get thirsty, we develop edema.

WAIT! I can't do this diet! Saliva tests? Tepid soup? Broccoli smoothies? One of the reasons I struggled with food for most of my life is that I like – love! – food. I want to enjoy being thin and that means enjoying **every** meal. And not treating my body like a chem lab experiment!

Is there some merit to the Dr. Atkins and other protein-based diets discussed in chapter four, the low-fat theory presented in chapter five and the Ph-balance diet presented above? Of course! There's some sense and some nonsense in each of them – and you can decide the ratio for yourself. You decide which theories and practices are best for you.

But now I hope you're ready to read in detail the SIMPLE, sound, easy, effective diet of my own creation.

It starts on the next page with one simple mantra:

Don't eat Flour!

Chapter Eight:
Why are we fat?

If you're like me, you've spent a lot of your life hiding. Hiding your weight under dark colors, vertical lines and strategically placed accessories to camouflage and draw attention away from lumps, bumps and bulges.

Maybe you've also hidden your weight through yo-yo dieting – never *really* fat for too long, never *really* thin for too long, so that your body type never settled permanently onto anyone's consciousness!

Master of Deception

More importantly, you've probably become a master of hiding the way you feel about your weight. Most of the people in your life – including your family and close friends – probably think you're a complacent size twelve or a comfortable size sixteen. You keep the dark thoughts, the feelings of guilt, failure and inadequacy buried under layers of smiles and well-managed cheer.

Unfortunately, we can't hide from the one person whose opinion matters most – our own. And the negative feelings about our weight affect all of our relationships -- with our lovers and spouses, our children and parents, our friends and coworkers. At some level, sometimes in ways in which we ourselves are unaware, we are plagued by self-doubt, the fear that we can't really do anything right if something as supposedly simple as maintaining a healthy weight eludes us.

I knew that what the diet industry was telling me was both contradictory and incomplete, and I felt comfortable, finally, using my mind, body and spirit as my personal diet consultant. But I didn't feel comfortable sharing this theory with other women without finding professional support.

This is why, even when I found a way of eating that worked for me – a proven way that's worked for half a decade – I continued to research books and talk to experts, seeking validation that eliminating flour was a sound dietary plan.

Give up Grains, Experts Agree

One of the experts I spoke with was C. Richard Mabray, M.D., a high-energy Texan whose expertise includes the treatment of obesity. Dr. Mabray is certified by The American Board of Bariatric Medicine, a certification board for physicians focused on the medical management of obesity through diet, exercise, behavioral modification and pharmacotherapy.

His clinical practice, located in Victoria, Texas includes treating obesity with low carbohydrate eating regimens. Dr. Mabray empowers his patients with tips on how to eat in a healthy low carb, high protein way and educates them with diet tips and eating habits for a lifetime of optimal health.

The first question I asked him: Why are so many Americans still fat?

His answer: processed grains, processed carbohydrates and processed fat.

"We didn't happen, we're made and the Lord told us back in Genesis 9 exactly what to eat and it hasn't changed in all of these thousands of years. He says, "OK guys, here's your human diet. You're gonna eat meat, fish and fowl. Well, I guess you could put snails and shrimp and other things in there but basically meat, fish and fowl and vegetables and he didn't mention grains and he didn't mention huge amounts of fruit or other processed things. And, obviously back in those days, the meat, fish and fowl were healthy, not penned up, fed out, fed with hormones, antibiotics, insecticides, pesticides, all the things that are hormone mimics and get us in trouble in that area."

It's past time, Dr. Mabray said, that the healthy diet pyramid is being re-examined."

"If it were a medicine, it would have been taken off the market a long time ago," Dr. Mabray said. "The American Heart Association diet should be called the American Heart Attack diet."

The medical community ignored the evidence – its own evidence – because they fell in love with their theory that a low-fat diet equaled low body fat. Dr. Mabray pointed to a study published in the National Geographic more than thirty years ago – January, 1973 – in which a community of long-lived residents – including a woman older than 130 – did all the "wrong" things, according to U.S. medical thinking. The evidence was so confusing, so contradictory (the residents also smoked!) that it was essentially ignored. The residents ate a lot of meat and drank a lot of water, a combination that has more recently been credited with health and lean body mass.

Dr. Mabray went on to say he advises patients to eliminate sugar (carbs), corn (grain), wheat (grain) and milk and to never skip meals if they want to get thin and stay thin.

He also tells them to avoid things that grow underground, such as potatoes, and that one of the problems with wheat (which includes flour) is that many people are allergic to gluten and, as I have found, we tend to become addicted to the foods that cause us the most trouble (flour products, milk, chocolate, etc.)

"When I do food testing, there is a very strong tendency – well over 75 percent – that people are allergic to the things they are addictively seeking. So, when we're allergic to a food, we tend to either hate it and avoid it like the plague or we addictively approach it. And so when I say milk, corn and wheat are not only bad actors for many reasons on their own, I also say this because obese people are allergic to them."

This makes sense to me. It certainly follows my pattern with pasta, with chocolate and, to some extent, even with fruit. If I eat too much fruit, I sort of start craving sweet things again. When I stick with protein and vegetables, I never feel compelled to overeat.

Internal Itch

Dr. Mabray compares the allergy/overeating symptom to an itch.

"It's like scratching an itch. When you quit scratching, if you can get past the scratch, then the itch will go away as the skin heals. It's an itch/scratch/itch kind of thing except this time it's an internal thing."

Dr. Mabray also supported my premise that all diets work to help you lose weight – the problem is that most diets don't help you keep weight off.

"When liquid and shake diets (a modified fast) were the in thing, people lost weight like mad," Dr. Mabray said. "It came off by the truckloads, but then they gained it all back faster than they took it off when they resumed eating. So, I think that in terms of weight loss, it's easy to see that all diets work if you work them, but the ones that work most effectively are those that limit carbohydrates and processed grains."

Dr. Mabray cited a study of 6000 men who had heart attacks. The men were put into three groups – a low fat group, a high fiber group and a group who ate three to five fish meals a week. The group that ate fish – the high protein, low carb group -- reduced the recurrence of heart attacks by thirty one percent, which is about the same reduction produced by drugs such as Lipitor™ and Pravachol™.

"It's the processed wheat and other grains that cause American's so many problems", Dr. Mabray explains. "I have a fantastic patient who grew up in France. She and her family rescued 22 downed Allied fliers during the war and got them into the French underground and back out. This woman would go back every summer and spend 2 or 3 months with her mother. She described a little bakery two blocks away from her mother's house where they baked with spelt, a different strain of wheat than the one we use, and the same yeast that had been in the family for 250 years. That's nutritionally very, very different from the wheat that we've got. We process our wheat so our bread puffs up quickly and easily when exposed to yeast. The processing of wheat and other grains destroys its nutritional value and ultimately leads to weight gain", Dr. Mabray said.

Dr. Mabray also supported Dr. Schwarzbein's concerns about insulin resistance and weight problems. "I find that virtually all people that are really struggling with weight that come see me are in some resistance. That means their cells are resistant to insulin and it takes more insulin for sugar to get into cells. If you are insulin resistant, you must eat more sugar for the insulin level to go up. You finally get the insulin and sugar levels high enough so that it works. But insulin is a growth hormone so it says 'OK, I've got to hold on to everything that comes in to protect me in the future.' So we get this vicious cycle, crave sugar, gain weight, can't lose, crave sugar, gain weight, can't lose."

This sugar craving, Dr. Mabray says, includes flour because all flour turns into sugar in the body. Flour and other grains are amylose sugars, not glucose. They are actually worse than pure sugar. It would be better to eat a teaspoon of sugar from the sugar bowl than to eat a piece of bread.

"Anyone who's struggling with weight should focus their diet on eating the things that are lower on the glycemic scale and stay away from those things that are high on the glycemic scale. And that means white flour, white rice, and processed corn."

I asked Dr. Mabray about exercise.

"People who exercise may counterbalance their insulin resistance. It's difficult to determine what constitutes enough physical activity to offset insulin resistance, but in other cultures and in earlier American history, most people had to be physically active. There weren't cars to take them everywhere, washing machines to take the labor out of laundry, and remote controls to eliminate even the minimal exercise of changing TV channels".

"I have a friend, an internal medicine doctor, who runs a clinic on the river by the Rio Grande. This is across the border from Texas and over the years, he's gone into the little villages, 20, 30 miles away to give residents vitamins and perform routine check-ups. Near the border, people are fat and they've got high blood pressure, their teeth are falling out, they've got diabetes, and they're sick. Now, their first cousins or brothers or sisters who live 30 miles away are all gorgeous. These people walk 10 or 15 miles to come see him and they're healthier because they have to walk everywhere.

They just walk. They don't run. They don't try to burn themselves up with iron man competition or jogging or things that are super-oxidating. They just walk and work. They work in the fields. They walk to town. They walk home and that's just a way of life for them. I think we've lost that."

I was glad to hear Dr. Mabray say this because for most of my years of gaining and losing weight, I would either exercise obsessively or not at all. I finally stopped because I hated it. I got a dog, and now I'm up walking at 6:30 every morning. It's saner and healthier. And, if you hate to exercise, Dr. Mabray has some other good news for you:

"There are some really good studies that show people who don't exercise lose weight easier than those who do exercise and that makes sense because if you're exercising, in my opinion "correctly", then you're going to gain muscle. It's the lifestyle exercise that really works. If people are forcing themselves to get to that fancy place to exercise, then they're going to run out of money or time, or cute gym clothes. You have to figure out what works for you. And it's the same with food. There are sensible diet principles, but it has to be their diet, not the Dr. Mabray diet. I think that's true with exercise as well. My prejudice is that healthy people that I see are those that have exercise as a lifestyle and are not obsessive about it. Excessive exercise burns people out and can cause injury and illness."

"I also believe that doctors don't know enough about nutrition to help their patients. The burden is passed onto dietitians, who are usually ill-equipped to sort out the hype from fact," Dr. Mabray said.

"Most of what they (doctors and dietitians) say, at least in my experience, is to rely on what the big grain companies tell them," Dr. Mabray said. "I have no proof of this, but I think the very origins of the American Dietary Association were funded and dreamed up by a coalition of big grain companies and the milk industry planning strategies to get more people to eat grain and milk"

The Opium Den of Milk and Wheat

Both milk and wheat, and wheat in contrast to other grains, produce a fairly dramatic number of breakdown products of addictive opiates. It requires special enzymes working correctly to be able to detoxify the body of those things.

Dr. Mabray said eating more protein is the best way to both end the grain and milk addiction because protein has a positive impact on insulin resistance, which produces the cravings. "It's important to reduce grains and other carbohydrates, Dr. Mabray said, and easier to resist them when more protein is included in the diet."

The average woman should get at least six ounces of protein "to make sure that insulin resistance isn't encouraged. It's a survival tool. And if you don't get the protein, the body thinks it's starving and so it slows down metabolism so you can live through the tough times."

If you eat six to eight ounces of protein at least three servings of vegetables and one or two servings of fruit a day, you will restrict grains and other carbohydrates naturally, Dr. Mabray said, without even bothering to count them.

No Grain/ No Pain

That's it! It was wonderful to get scientific support for my intuitive findings about permanent weight loss. I also liked that Dr. Mabray provided evidence to say that giving up our grain addictions can be simplified by adding protein to our diets. A chicken wing could be your anti-flour patch (to eat, not apply to your shoulder!) and chewing a piece of steak could be the dietary equivalent to nicotine gum.

When you treat your body the way it was meant to be treated, it naturally protects you from the evil effects of grains and other carbohydrates. When you eat more protein, you lose the addictive cravings. Isn't it nice to know that eating not just one but an entire bag of Hershey's kisses is not because you lack willpower but because you are feeding a chemically-controlled addiction? And isn't it even nicer – ecstatic – that you can beat the addiction by replacing carb-laden foods with protein-rich foods?

Still not convinced? Well, since I'm staking my reputation – and your thinness – on the no-grain philosophy, I promise you more proof in the next chapter.

Why are we fat?

Flour and starchy carbs bad. Protein good.

Dr. Mabray made it sound so simple and his views were so reaffirming that it was tempting to stop my research right there. Tempting but unfair to you. After all, I'm asking you to change your eating habits – your life – forever, and you deserve to know how well the experts support (or refute) my views. So I spent some time with Dr. Shoshana Zimmerman, co-author of *My Doctor Says I'm Fine, So Why do I Feel so Bad?*

I began by asking her the same question I asked Dr. Mabray: Why are we so fat?

Dr. Zimmerman, a doctor of naturopathy with an office in Palo Alto, California, said that some people simply eat too much junk food. Plain and simple. But what's not so simple is that people who do not overeat but who eat processed carbohydrates, such as flour, also gain (or are unable to lose) weight because they have an extra sensitivity to them.

"Food sensitivities and even environmental sensitivities can prevent weight loss. Flour is one of the most common things that people are sensitive to and when they are sensitive to it, they find it impossible to lose weight," Dr. Zimmerman said. Additionally, they may also feel congested and suffer from other symptoms.

Dr. Zimmerman said it is possible to be tested for carbohydrate sensitivity. She recommends that anyone who has excess mucous get a blood test called IGG antibody test.

Dr. Zimmerman said an allergist will test for IGG, a kind of blood test that will show if you have an out-and-out allergy (passing out, can't breathe, get hives, start sneezing coughing, etc.) But the IGG antibody test also shows when a person has a very slow carbohydrate sensitivity building up.

"For example, a person could have been eating wheat their whole life and one day wake up and they can't have wheat any more. They start having an allergy reaction. They have passed sensitivity to allergy."

"Most people never pass over that line into allergy, they just stay sensitive and they don't know what it is, they just complain about their symptoms. And if gluten is involved, and the gluten is not just wheat but corn and barley and other products, it can lead to obesity and diabetes."

Refined carbohydrates, such as flour, release sugar rapidly into a person's bloodstream. When you get a fast release of those sugars the body takes the flour and converts it into sugar and when that hits your body really fast then you get a spike.

"That spike will give you a good energy sensation for a while and then it will dip. The reason for this is that insulin will stop trying to convert the sugar into energy. Or, if it cannot be used up in energy because the person has a sedentary lifestyle or they're having too many carbs and they don't need all that energy, it gets converted into fat. That conversion, over a long period of time, slowly increases cholesterol and triglycerides. This is why people can be on a low fat diet and put on weight if they're eating high carbs."

Dr. Zimmerman said a person's ability to use carbs without gaining weight depends on body type. She uses the Eastern, Ayurveda philosophy to distinguish body types.

Carb-Friendly Batas

The first is the model type, the long-legged person. This body type can usually consume more carbs than others. "They're very light and they tend to be very active. They've moving around all the time, hence the build. They have what's called high bata energy. They need a little bit of extra heaviness so they tend to do well eating carbs without having the kinds of problems that other body types have. They're not as sensitive to it. But even they, if they go on a junk food diet for a long period of time - their shape's going to change."

The Medium Build Pittas

The second body type, Dr. Zimmerman said, is called pitta. "These are the people who have a really medium frame. They're not big. They're not skinny. They're not long. They're not tall. They're not short. They tend to be take-charge types. They always have a to-do list. They have a lot of digestive energy. They metabolize things very well and so, they also tend to be active and as long as they can have a sense of control in their life, and not be overwhelmed with too much stress, they can have great metabolic function. They too can have a large number of carbs and burn it up with minimal bad side effects. As long as they don't get too sedentary and they don't eat high carbs over a long period of time. They will, however be likely to start very slowly but surely putting on the weight over a 10, 20, 30 year period of high carb eating.

Caution to Kaphas and Bobosas

The third type is called kapha, Dr. Zimmerman said. "They're the ones with the hourglass figures, smaller waists, big hips and they have enormous stamina but they tend to have slow digestion. They have thick bones. They're the ones who can fall down. They don't get bone problems. They don't get osteoporosis easily. They have to really have horrible diets to get osteoporosis but they have very slow digestion. And these people, even on a small amount of carbs have problems. These are your prime candidates for pancreatic insufficiency. (It's the pancreas that releases the insulin.) These types get tired, they reach for a Coke or coffee or a sugar snack because they are tired.

Then there's the bobasa. (I swear this was me!)

"A bobasa type starts living primarily on carbs because they think it's healthier. So they're eating bagels and they're eating salads and they're having lots of pasta and hardly any fat. And they work out all the time. They will complain to you that they have fat on their legs, on their thighs that they can't get rid of even though they eat healthy and exercise all the time. They can't get rid of their bellies - meaning that at some point their belly was flatter - even though they do a zillion crunches. They won't get rid of it because when carbs are excessive, even with the burning of more calories, it starts storing fat there."

"When this gets out of control, the waist will thicken and these women really start putting it on from the breast to the hips. They are the ones in greatest danger. They're the ones that are most likely to develop diabetes."

What's a Kapha to do?

Dr. Zimmerman says kapha people who are especially sensitive to foods will usually have problems with anything containing sugar. For kapha types who want the dietary benefits of fruit, Dr. Zimmerman recommends the tarter variety, such as strawberries and warns against sweet fruits such as watermelon. Her book details the foods to eat and avoid according to body type.

Other examples include the fact that high-fiber fruits take longer to digest and are better for insulin-resistant persons. On the other hand, fruit juice metabolizes quickly (like refined flour), so that a person who eats a bagel and drinks a glass of juice might find themselves nodding out an hour or so later."

Body type really makes a difference in the way a person processes food.

Energy Code

At the point of conception, Dr. Zimmerman said, everyone gets an energy code, just as they get a DNA code. When a person stays in balance for her body type, all is well. When a person gets out of balance, trouble arises. Anyone can gain weight if they get out of balance by replacing their regular meals with junk foods.

The degree of balance (or imbalance) can be tested. Dr. Zimmerman said it shows up in the pulse. She said she feels fifty six pulses in each of a person's arms and measures the difference between the two. And when a person is in balance, the cravings for the foods that put them out of balance disappear. This explains, then, why my flour cravings have disappeared.

If anyone had told me five years ago that I could live without flour – happily – I would have told them they were crazy. I never really understood why I didn't have the cravings to satisfactorily explain them to anyone. Now I know, thanks to Dr. Zimmerman and others, that there really is a biochemical explanation. Flour was the food that put me most out of balance. Once I eliminated it from my diet and regained balance, I lost all desire for it. Dr. Zimmerman said food that's right for you restores the intestinal wall (if you want to look it up, it's called *agglutinin*) and – ta da! – reduces sugar cravings.

It all makes sense! Even better – it works! Giving up flour has been the smartest, most successful diet strategy of my life, and I believe it can be just as powerful for you.

A Commitment to Be Thin

So what did I take from the Atkins diet? The fact that I need to reduce carbs to about 60 grams a day to lose weight and **slightly** more to maintain weight. Easiest way to do that is to stop eating foods that have the highest carb count – flour – and eat more protein instead.

...And from the low fat, heart-healthy proponents? I need to be smart about how much and the type of fats I eat. High fat means high calorie. If I stay away from flour, I am also staying away from processed high fat foods such as crackers, cookies, cakes, pastries,

etc. These fats are definitely bad and high in calories that my somewhat sedentary body is just dying to store.

...And from the Raw diet? Eat my vegetables and fruits. My body needs the benefits of the complex carbs and the energy that they provide.

As a result, I began winning my last war on weight when I followed through on this very simple plan:

- Don't eat any flour.
- Eat six to eight ounces of protein, at least three big servings of vegetables and one or two servings of fruit a day.
- Enjoy a nice glass of red wine, but make it a 4oz. glass 2-3 times a week.
- Don't skip meals and add a morning and evening snack.
- Stay committed by focusing in on that mind, body, spirit connection. You don't need to weigh yourself to know if you are bringing about the change you desire. You will feel it and be elated by that feeling. Only weigh yourself once every month, anything more is as bad as eating a bagel.

For me, the commitment to give up flour is a realistic and easy rule in an effort to control all the other unhealthy no-nos: **bad fats, refined sugar, bad carbs & high calories.**

Simple, right? Wrong! It's one of the toughest transitions I've ever made. The commitment to change my weight and my relationship with food once and for all worked – and continues to work seven years later.

Now, I'm going to help you do the same. Are you ready to make that personal commitment? If you are, you can begin your final journey toward permanent weight loss right now - starting with the Ten Commitments.

Part Three:

Light at the End of the Tunnel

Chapter Nine:
The Ten Commitments

The First Commitment
Don't Even Go There!

The supermarket is a challenge to a diet. When I go food shopping, I stay out of the aisles and do my shopping on the outer perimeters. Why? Because that is where "my food" is plentiful without having to contemplate the crackers, cookies, snacks, and the quick fix, easy, gazillions of prepared foods that prey on my "gotta have it now" style of eating. When you give up flour, you give up the need to contemplate ALL prepared foods. No more staring at a box of Entenmann's and wondering, "Hmmmm, maybe….." There are no flour carbs to count – they are OUT!

Be sure the allowed foods (lean protein, veggies, fruits, nuts and dairy) are readily and quickly available for snacking. And please –stay away from potatoes and other chips! You don't need the empty calories and the fat. Remember this is your relationship. You are choosing it. No one is watching.

The Second Commitment
Never Take the First Bite

I have found nirvana in that the only way to get rid of the dense, starchy carb cravings is to not have any at all. The kind you find in flour such as breads, pasta, cakes, cookies, crackers, cereals, etc. It takes time, but every day the carb cravings lessen, and my cravings for fresh fruit, veggies and lean protein heighten.

I know what you're saying… "This broad is tapped! Why can't I have a piece of light wheat bread? It's only forty calories and nine grams of carbs." You can! You can do whatever you want. All of this is a choice. I only know in my experience of gaining and losing hundreds of pounds that a bite- turns into a slice -- turns into a loaf. Why put yourself through that misery when all you have to commit to is not taking the first bite?

The Third Commitment
Engage Your Imagination

Okay, any trick, gimmick or delusion can be your genius when it comes to controlling what you eat. When I am in a situation where fabulous appetizers and gorgeous desserts are just under my nose, I set my mind to a place, where it always is after I indulge.

Where's the pleasure? It's in your mouth and then it's gone. All that lingers is the memory of what it tasted like, and guilt. But if

I imagine that I just ate it-I end up in the same place. I remember what it tasted like, but with no guilt.

Practice this and suddenly, you're free of making the agonizing decision: to have-or not to have. Because you already devoured it, and now you can move on!

The Fourth Commitment
Buy a George Foreman Grill

One common trait we overeaters share is the tendency to grab the quickest, easiest 'gotta have it now' foods, especially during stressful days.

Instead of trying to completely change my natural eating tendencies, I changed my roster of 'gotta have it now' comfort foods. (ie: nuts, instead of chips or goldfish; strawberries and low fat cheese instead of M&Ms; a cup of coffee with light cream and an apple instead of coffee with skim milk and chocolate chip cookies.)

Get creative with healthy fast food lunches and dinners. This is where the George Foreman Grill became my diet partner. It is the most essential tool for maintaining my eating lifestyle because it is a fast and easy solution.

For example, you can freeze a bag of chicken breasts, take a couple out as you need them, pre heat the George Foreman for a few minutes, throw them on the grill frozen, time for 7-8 minutes, go away, come back when you hear the timer and they are ready to eat!

George Foreman is portable – you can even bring your grill to the office, prepare your lunches there and enjoy great, flour-free meals every day.

This is especially effective during the day when I usually only have fifteen minutes for lunch. I take that grilled chicken breast and put it over a Caesar Salad or some other creative salad with grilled chicken or fish, lots of veggies and/or fruit and low fat cheese.

The Fifth Commitment
Don't Ever Say Diet

I can hear you now. "I read about (yet another) *this diet* where you give up flour. So I'm giving *this diet* a shot."

Make no mistake about it, this is not a 'diet'. This is an adjustment to your eating style. This is a major overhaul in your relationship with food. It is composed, crafted and tested by you, because no expert knows better than you what makes you fatter than you want to be. Is it dense starchy carbs? What kind? Pasta, Subs, Bagels?

Okay - stay away, they're trigger foods. That's the whole program in two words NO FLOUR, if you have determined by this stage of the book that flour is, without a doubt, your trigger food.

Remove the trigger, remove the addicted reaction to food. Stay away from the foods that compel you to overeat, and you never have to take a course in ph-balance or keep a dipstick in your purse.

The Sixth Commitment
Get Creative

Be creative with your food! I only learned to cook when I threw away the recipe books (and the pasta) and started to experiment by putting anything that would go on bread or pasta - onto a salad. Learn to have fun creating wonderful dishes using your favorite 'allowed' foods. I can honestly say that I love food more now because I've put a stop to the love/hate relationship that drove my eating habits.

Before, the only thing I knew how to cook was pasta dishes and sandwiches, anything else was a lot of effort and took too long. Try getting creative. No recipes. Just your personal tastes as guidance. See what you come up with. These are a few of mine.

Most of these recipes are for single servings:

Ricotta cheese with warm apples

1/2c fat free ricotta cheese

1 medium apple cored and sliced into large chunks

dash cinnamon

1 Tbsp. honey roasted soy nuts, walnuts or almonds

Place apple chunks and nuts in small microwave safe bowl. Add cinnamon. Microwave on high for 2-3 minutes until apples are juicy and tender.

Remove and let cool for 5 minutes.

Top off with chilled ricotta cheese and enjoy!

(You can substitute ricotta cheese with fat free cottage cheese or plain, non-fat yogurt. You can also substitute apples for chilled pineapple chunks in its own juice, blueberries or strawberries.)

Grilled Chicken Pesto Salad with Sun Dried Tomatoes and Broccoli

2c. Lettuce

3-4 oz. warm, grilled chicken tenders or breast sliced (sauté in a splash of olive oil, balsamic vinegar, garlic and fresh basil to taste)

2 Tbsp. sundried tomatoes in oil

1-2 Tbsp. pesto (Try Buittoni's reduced fat pesto with basil)

8-10 sweet grape tomatoes

Fresh broccoli florets, steamed until tender, but not mushy

1 Tbsp. pine nuts (optional)

2 Tbsp. shredded light mozzarella cheese

Place chilled lettuce into a large salad bowl. (A pasta bowl works best!)

Toss with pesto and sun dried tomatoes. (Drain most of the oil from the tomatoes, leaving a small amount to moisten and flavor the lettuce)

Add grape tomatoes, broccoli and pine nuts

Top off with chicken

Sprinkle with mozzarella cheese

Seafood or Tuna Salad with Grapes and Walnuts

2c. Lettuce

3-4 oz. seafood salad (you can get from your supermarket deli)

10 seedless red grapes

2-3 Tbsp. walnuts, chopped

Olive oil & balsamic vinegar to taste

Place chilled lettuce into a large salad bowl. (A pasta bowl works best!)

Toss in olive oil and balsamic vinegar.

Add grapes and walnuts. Top off with seafood salad and enjoy!

Grilled Chicken with Apples, Dried Cranberries, Goat Cheese and Pecan

2c. Lettuce

3-4 oz. warm, grilled chicken tenders or breast sliced (sauté in a splash of olive oil, balsamic vinegar, garlic and fresh basil to taste)

1/2 apple, sliced (sweet, such as gala or empire)

2 Tbsp. dried cranberries

2 Tbsp. crumpled goat cheese

2 Tbsp. pecans, chopped or whole

Chopped onion to taste

(Try Emeril's Orange Herb with Poppy Seeds Marinade and Salad Dressing available in most supermarkets)

Place chilled lettuce into a large salad bowl. (A pasta bowl works best!)

Toss in salad dressing

Add apples, cranberries and goat cheese

Place chicken slices on top (optional)

Sprinkle with whole or chopped pecans

Grilled Veggies

When weather permits, grilling is a fabulous tool. Why? Number one, no dirty pots and pans. Number two, you can get your husband to do the cooking. Number three, it's essentially a healthier way to cook.

Here is one of my favorite grilled veggie dishes.

Chop the following vegetables into large pieces and place in a large bowl:

1 Green pepper

1 Red pepper

1 Yellow zucchini

1 c. cubed turnip (parboil first)

1 Apple (cut into ½ inch wedges)

2 Tbsp. Olive Oil

1 Tsp. each of garlic powder, apple pie spice and pepper

Dash salt

Sprinkle olive oil over the mixture. Add Garlic powder, salt, pepper and apple pie spice to taste. Mix together

Place the tossed mixture into a grilling basket and grill for about twenty-five minutes or until desired tenderness. Choose medium heat on a gas grill. Close the lid on the grill and toss the mixture every few minutes. Cook until tender.

Mashed Cauliflower

Stop mourning mashed potatoes. These taste just as great – without the weight!

Chop up a full head of cauliflower florets into smallish pieces

Parboil OR put in a microwave safe dish with 2-3 Tbsp. water and a Tsp. of minced garlic.

(steam or microwave until tender/soft) When you can stick a fork through the florets easily, they're done!

Drain. Put the florets in food processor. Add ¼ to ½ c. Fat-Free Half and Half and a Tbsp. of butter or butter substitute. Puree until mashed potato consistency.

Add salt and pepper to taste. Enjoy!

Simple and Simply Incredible Chicken

1 Chicken breast – boneless, skinless

2 Tbsp. Olive oil

1 Tbsp. Chopped or minced garlic

1 red or green pepper (cut in large pieces)

½ c. black olives (cut in half)

4 artichoke hearts (canned in water)

10-12 grape tomatoes (cut in half)

2 c. fresh spinach

Saute chicken breast about eight minutes in a splash of olive oil and garlic. Add pepper, olives, artichoke hearts and grape tomatoes, let all that simmer together until vegetables are tender. Add fresh spinach. Cover. Let simmer until the spinach is wilted and at desired tenderness. Voila – a whole meal. Serve it with the mashed cauliflower, and it's fabulous!!

Pecan encrusted ANYTHING

Just because you're giving up flour doesn't mean you have to give up the crunchiness of flour-coated fried foods. Here's a way to add great taste and a bunch of crunch without guilt. My example uses chicken breasts, but you could use this to coat any meat or fish. I like this with tuna, salmon and haddock.

Chop about a cup of pecans in a food processor until they reach a fine (breadcrumb-like) consistency. Beat an egg. Dip the chicken into the egg and roll it into pecans. (You can substitute olive oil for the egg if you like). Bake in a 350-degree oven for about 30 minutes – or until done to desired tenderness. You can use any kind of nuts you prefer such as walnuts, cashews, etc. Try flavoring the mixture with Amaretto, vanilla or orange flavoring.

Baked Apple with Walnuts

1 large apple (I recommend Cortland) cored
1 Tsp. Apple pie spice
1/2 Tbsp. butter (It is best to substitute Smart Balance, I Can't Believe Its Not Butter, etc.)

6-7 walnuts whole or chopped

2-3 Tbsp. Light Cool Whip

Place cored apple in an oven safe shallow dish.

Fill the hollowed core with walnuts and butter.

Sprinkle with Apple pie spice.

Bake at 350 for about 40 minutes or until VERY juicy and tender.

Remove and let cool.

Smother with chilled or slightly frozen cool whip and indulge!

Orange and Raspberry Jell-O Parfait

1 blood or navel orange sectioned and then cut into medium size chunks

1 c. sugar free raspberry Jell-O (already prepared and chilled)

2-3 Tbsp. Light Cool Whip

Spoon half of the Jell-O into a parfait dish.

Add a layer of orange chunks.

Add another layer of Jell-O.

Finish with the remaining orange chunks.

Top off with Cool Whip and enjoy!

Favorite Snack Plate

A few slices of Cabot's 75% reduced fat cheddar cheese

6 or 7 apple slices

1/4 c. mixed nuts lightly salted or salt free

The Seventh Commitment
Realize this is a Choice

When you decide to diet, you immerse yourself in some God-awful rigid set of eating do's and don'ts. You resent the fact that this is what it will take to lose weight, because that is what one diet guru or another nutrition expert says is your path to losing weight.

You're on your own path. If you don't like it, change it. It's a choice, one only you can make.

When you are making decisions about which foods to eat and which to eliminate heed the understanding that you are choosing your relationship with food. One that will lead to the body you will ultimately have. Staying away from flour, making smart choices about fats and eliminating starchy vegetables, such as potatoes, to once a week in small doses – are the food choices that give me the body I have today.

The Eighth Commitment
Listen to Your Body, Mind, Spirit

I'm not disputing that most of these popular diets make you lose weight. You've already proven that with the many pounds you've lost. But what about maintaining your weight loss and all that goes with it? What about that body, mind, spirit connection that happens, when you are committed to something that you are passionate about?

Like the empowered attitude, stronger commitment and an unwavering belief in your ability to reach your goals. Keep tapping into that glorious feeling. It will drive your steel resolve and generate strength for your journey ahead. Remember, once you gravitate back to your trigger foods, as you have in the past or you wouldn't be reading this book, you gain weight and lose that body, mind and spirit connection.

The Ninth Commitment
Forgive Yourself

For much of your life, you've been a victim of your self-criticism as much as you've been a victim of food cravings, diet programs or fashion magazines.

Eat one bite of "forbidden" food and we replay every bad movie our minds have produced. We don't feel guilty about one chocolate chip cookie. We berate ourselves for every food "mistake" we've ever made, every dress we couldn't squeeze into, every exercise program we didn't complete and, while we're at it, we criticize ourselves for every promotion we didn't get, homework assignment we didn't complete and parental expectation we didn't meet.

We're good at the guilt – so good that it undermines many – sometimes all – of our progress.

Forgive yourself NOW for every pound you've gained or failed to lose in the past and any misstep you might make in the future. Reward yourself for every step forward, no matter how small. Reward yourself today for finding the path that will lead you to achieving your weight loss goals.

The Tenth Commitment
Commit for Today

Before I decided to make this commitment, if anyone told me that I could lose all the weight I wanted with just one simple commitment: Give up any foods made with flour for the rest of my life, I would have thought it impossible.

Today, I still think it impossible- to fathom the rest of my life without foods that I love, much the way you are feeling.

But if I ask you, "Could you give it up for today if it meant losing and maintaining the healthy weight you want to be?"

Of course you can and you would want to make that commitment.

Only for today.

Tomorrow you can do whatever you wish, but the change comes about by making the commitment for today.

Screw tomorrow. Tomorrow is another day.

Chapter Ten:
Flour-free Foodstyles

Whether you attend four charity functions a week, travel for business six times a month or spend most of your waking and sleeping hours at home, you can easily manage your commitment to a flour-free life.

I know this because I've kept up my flour-free ways during all manner of personal and professional transitions. Whether I'm dining in heels at a four-star restaurant or barefoot at home with my four-legged friends, I make healthy, tasty choices every day.

And to show you how you can do it, too, I've categorized lifestyles into food "groupies". (Hey don't snicker. We've all been there as food worshipers at one point or another!)

- Super (market) models – women who eat most of their meals at home because of family and/or job commitments.
- Men(u) Pleasers – women who conduct business (and must eat) at restaurants.
- Buff(et) Beauties – women who attend charity functions or other banquet-style meal events.
- McD(amsels)—women who dine frequently at fast-food restaurants.

Super (market) models

Stick to the rim. Most, if not all, of the food you can buy (and eat!) without guilt will be located on the perimeter of the store. Fill your basket with items from the produce, dairy and meat departments. Venture into the middle aisles ONLY if you are looking for a specific item (such as spices or olive oil) and return to the rim immediately. (Because if you linger near the cinnamon sticks too long you are likely to get (a) hungry and (b)tempted to grab a box of cinnamon rolls located ever-so-conveniently near the spice rack.)

Some tips for making your grocery list: think about buying the best possible of everything. If you're buying mushrooms, for instance, handpick some button mushrooms instead of grabbing a ready-made carton. Or try different kinds of mushrooms – portabella, for instance – and experiment with greens. Try snap peas instead of celery, Vidalia onions instead of a generic yellow onion, spinach instead of your usual lettuce. Most of us are creatures of habit, but if you get too bored with your food choices, you are likely to seek excitement from the wrong food aisles. So before you wander off into the forbidden cookie-and-cake zones, ask the produce clerk to let you sample a fruit you've never tried – a mango, maybe or perhaps a persimmon? You can awaken your taste buds – and sedate your food cravings quite enjoyably this way.

Practice creativity in all "good" areas of the grocery store. If you've only eaten canned tuna, try fresh. If you usually pick up a package of chicken breasts, try turkey breasts instead. Consider buying tiny amounts of six different kinds of fish or seafood and grilling on skewers. Have fun.

When you reach the dairy aisle, stock up on low-fat cheeses. If you want to mix in some richer choices, buy them in small quantities and experiment. If you purchase from the deli counter, you can buy a slice at a time. This way, if you end up with something you don't like, you don't waste money – and if you buy something you love, you're not tempted to eat the whole pound. Try farmer's cheese or fat free ricotta cheese instead of cottage cheese to mix with fruit or experiment with different plain, non-fat yogurt brands and textures to use in vegetable dips, soups and stews. Don't let your food choices become boring and you won't miss the grains.

Men(u) Pleasers

First rule: refuse the bread basket. If you're not *absolutely* ready to give up dough-y delights, you can follow Ellen's rule. She asks the waiter to deliver the bread basket at the end of the meal. Most often, she forgets or the waiter does, and she leaves the table bread-free. If the server brings the basket and she can't resist a bite or two of a roll, well, she eats a bite or two – no more. Gone are her days of ordering a second basket before the meal.

Second rule: Don't read the pasta portion of the menu – it doesn't exist for you. From the rest of the menu, however, you should find plenty of tasty, healthy non-flour choices.

Third rule: If you want the kitchen to change something for you and don't want to bring "diet" into the conversation, try saying "I'm allergic to…" It ALWAYS works, whether the chef is genuinely concerned or the owner is afraid of a lawsuit. But if you want "fried" chicken, try saying you're allergic to wheat – can you get your food pecan-crusted instead? If not pecan-crusted, then prepared in another way. If you ask politely, you can get almost anything.

If you eat out regularly, you will find it easy to order what's right for you, whether it's on or off the menu. In some ways, the infrequent restaurant patron has it harder. For her, a restaurant is sort of like a vacation – when the rules of self-discipline (including diet) disappear. If you ONLY eat out twice a year, you can probably get away with this lapse. But if you eat out more than once a month, don't be fooled by your own illogic. Enjoy the restaurant experience – the ambience and healthy food choices – so you leave with pleasant memories and not a doggie bag of regret.

Buff(et) Beauties

Buffet dining is really pretty easy – if you can avoid temptation. There are plenty of choices, so head for the salads and the meats – and don't try convincing yourself that if you eat a slice of cake standing up, it doesn't count!! You know better!

Be smart about what you put on your plate – and go ahead and make a second trip to the buffet. Yes, you can eat too much of *anything*, but it's really, really hard to eat too much lettuce or too much chicken (and you can't say the same for potato chips or pie).

McD(amsels)

Give the fast-food restaurants their due – most are trying to offer healthier, carb-reduced selections on their menus. If McDonald's can put lettuce-wraps on their menu, the least you can do is choose them – or an equally healthy selection instead of a burger on a bun. You aren't *required* to order French fries and no one will force you to buy the two-for-a-dollar apple pies. Although some drive-through restaurants are more diet-friendly than others, it is possible to keep the no-flour pledge anywhere you go. When it comes to grains, just say no! EVERY fast food restaurant offers meat and nearly every drive-through includes salad on their menus. So, yes, you CAN get fat eating at fast-food places, but it's not their fault if you do.

Bottom line: once you decide that flour doesn't exist in your world, you will stop seeing it in grocery stores or on menus. Your eyes, your brain and, yes, even your taste buds, will naturally gravitate to the 'good' foods, the foods that are right for you.

Just one warning: Don't fall victim to the "lower net carb" trap. You will find this on the menus that sell very HIGH CARB items such as bagels or on television commercials for cereal. There is no such thing as a low-carb bread or grain product. They don't exist.

And what's with the "net carb"? This new bit of marketing magic does not remove any carbohydrates from a bagel, and I wouldn't trust my weight loss to it. Marketers are not your dieting friends. Beware tricky language that will add pounds to both your "net" and "gross" weights.

Chapter Eleven:
Welcome to My World

Imagine a world in which there is no such thing as flour. No breads, pasta, cereals, cakes, cookies, pastries, pretzels or bagels. Now imagine your most decadent cravings are for apples, oranges, nuts, and cheese with a nice glass of red wine. Imagine guilt-free eating.

You will have this delicious lifestyle -- filled with healthy habits and absolutely zero cravings for foods that simply do not exist in my – and now your – world.

You will experience what I've experienced over the last few years. Seeing Atkins come, go and come again, seeing the marketing go from low-fat to adding thousands of new carb-friendly choices, you will no longer be victimized by these claims. It is incredibly empowering to NEVER have to deal with diet ads, to never feel a sense of diet information overload when scanning magazine covers or flipping through TV commercials. At one time I felt completely compelled to know about every weight loss claim and I focused on all of those messages. Now, I look at the magazine covers, and the headlines don't apply to me any more. I don't have to be concerned about how to drop seven pounds in seven days, or which celebrity just dropped a dress size on which diet. I don't need to DIET any more, and, if you give up grains, neither will you!

Essentially, my food choices are low-carb, but that isn't the be-all and end-all to my belief system. I do believe that there is a difference between good and bad carbohydrates – the carbs in broccoli and the carbs in a donut are not created equally. I also don't believe that low-carb means returning to a high fat diet, particularly saturated fat. I'm not going to start eating bacon by the pound because it contains no carbohydrates. Come on! I've seen what bacon fat looks like in the pan, and I really don't want that kind of fat running (or slogging) through my veins.

It's also vital that you take your lifestyle into consideration. One of the reasons the high-carb diet SEEMED to work is that it coincided with the fitness craze. People who run five miles a day will burn carbohydrates (and may need them for fuel), but I don't run five miles, or even five blocks a day. Do you?

I exercise, yes, but am I at the gym every day? No. I love yoga, pilates and weight-training, but do I do any of these consistently? No, I can't always count on that. I DO walk my dogs three times a day, and I CAN count on that! I can also count on the fact that I'm always going to be a high-energy person who wakes up at seven a.m. – no matter what. I can count on maintaining a reasonably active lifestyle and planning a diet based on these realities.

I can always count on the fact that eating natural foods such as fruits, vegetables, low-fat dairy and lean proteins are always going to be the healthiest choices – and no diet trend ever disputes that.

(Some marketers will try to fool you into thinking that packaged food is equally good.) I can count on my history of being healthy and happy with my food relationship for the last seven years. I can take comfort in the fact that I haven't had a cold in the last three or four years.

Can I PROVE that my eating style is directly responsible for that? NO. Maybe it's a combination of what my body is taking in and the body, mind, spirit connection that I've maintained. Perhaps I'm feeding that healthy attitude. But I also know that for all of my adult life – all of my flour-filled adult life -- I had a severe cold at the beginning of every winter, and then several would follow. Since I became flour-free, I haven't had a single cold or flu – without a flu shot.

Here's another great thing: as I write this, I'm approaching my fiftieth birthday and I love it! For the first time in years, I don't need to be wearing designer clothes to feel attractive or to impress anyone with a fancy label. I'm happy with a $15 pair of jeans and a $10 t-shirt because I know when I slip them on, I'm going to look great. Thanks to a flour-free lifestyle, I'm at a comfortable body weight. That's the gift that my commitment has given me.

Trust me, I remember what it was like to be unable to trust myself with food. There was a time that, left to my own devices, I could have destroyed myself with either eating and gaining weight or binging and throwing up. I was a candidate for the most severe weight-related problems because I was OUT OF CONTROL with food. I would go to extremes to either satisfy my addiction or alleviate my guilt.

Giving up flour restored my control over food and this control gives me enormous freedom. My self-image, my pant size, my relationships, my career path ARE NOT defined by food. Giving up flour released me from a lifelong, debilitating dependency on the starchy, high calorie, high carb foods that were at the root of my misery.

I enjoy the freedom that we all seek. The freedom to know we're making the right choices and are not following the path of greatest pull or least resistance. With billions of dollars behind the experts who communicate health and nutrition information, I found no other way to have that freedom. When I decided I was done with flour – done with it – I gained control and lost excess weight for good. Amazing, but true. When I found a way to stop allowing food to control me, I also stopped being controlled by other forces.

Another amazing benefit – I enjoy eating now more than I ever had, and I've discovered I'm a very creative cook. I feel the freedom to be inventive, to not follow recipes. I experiment, make things up – and voila – I've got another great dish! So, don't overwhelm yourself looking for flour-free recipes. Make them up as you go along. That's the fun of it – the freedom. Remove one obstacle from your life – and add so much more.

I did not invent a 'diet'– the talk shows are full of doctors who do more than enough of that. Instead, I went Against The Grain. I'm an average woman who discovered she's not-so-average in mid-life. I gave up self-doubt and unburied my passions, putting both talent and skill to personal and professional purpose. When you give up on your self- doubt, you, too, will connect with your brilliance. Another thing, for as long as I was controlled by food, I didn't trust in my intellect. How could a smart woman be overweight when she wanted so badly to be thin? Could a savvy woman be gullible enough to believe in grapefruit diets? As long as I was that overweight, food-controlled woman, I couldn't find the confidence to change other areas of my life. I want to connect with women who feel the same way, and that's why I'm writing this book – to lift you, the reader, onto a platform of hope. By establishing a healthy relationship with food, I know you will find a lot more.

You, too, can take the no-flour path to a delicious and fulfilling lifestyle, and I want to nurture and share in your success. Please email me at againstgrain@comcast.net, and tell me how you are achieving your goals. Your story can reach out to others just as mine has to you. No one knows your relationship with food the way you do. Use my experience as a guidepost and my success as inspiration, but chart your own course.

Just make sure you are honest with yourself. I understand if you don't want to confess to your husband that you – and not the dog – polished off three jelly donuts in the middle of the night. But don't try to fool yourself with such powder-sugared lies. When I came to terms with the fact that I can't control my flour intake – *it controls me* – and opted it out of my life forever, I was choosing honesty over deception.

So, create YOUR path, the one that works for you, the one that will become YOUR lifelong permanent weight maintenance program. Be kind – and honest – with yourself if you make an occasional wrong choice. Get over it, reconnect with your magnificence and get on with your life!

Food		Calories	Carbs
1000 ISLAND, SALAD DRSNG,LOCAL	1 TBSP	25	2
1000 ISLAND, SALAD DRSNG,REGLR	1 TBSP	60	2
100% NATURAL CEREAL	1 OZ	35	18
40% BRAN FLAKES, KELLOGG'S	1 OZ	90	22
40% BRAN FLAKES, POST	1 OZ	90	22
ALFALFA SEEDS, SPROUTED, RAW	1 CUP	10	1
ALL-BRAN CEREAL	1 OZ	70	21
ALMONDS, SLIVERED	1 CUP	795	28
ALMONDS, WHOLE	1 OZ	165	6
ANGELFOOD CAKE, FROM MIX	1 CAKE	1510	342
ANGELFOOD CAKE, FROM MIX	1 PIECE	125	29
APPLE JUICE, CANNED	1 CUP	115	9
APPLE PIE	1 PIE	2420	360
APPLE PIE	1 PIECE	405	60
APPLESAUCE, CANNED, SWEETENED	1 CUP	195	51
APPLESAUCE, CANNED,UNSWEETENED	1 CUP	105	28
APPLES, DRIED, SULFURED	10 RINGS	155	42
APPLES, RAW, PEELED, SLICED	1 CUP	65	16
APPLES, RAW, UNPEELED,2 PER LB	1 APPLE	125	32
APPLES, RAW, UNPEELED,3 PER LB	1 APPLE	80	21
APRICOT NECTAR, NO ADDED VIT C	1 CUP	140	36
APRICOTS, CANNED, JUICE PACK	1 CUP	120	31
APRICOTS, CANNED, JUICE PACK	3 HALVES	40	10
APRICOTS, DRIED, COOKED,UNSWTN	1 CUP	210	55
APRICOTS, DRIED, UNCOOKED	1 CUP	310	80
APRICOTS, RAW	3 APRCOT	50	12
APRICOT, CANNED, HEAVY SYRUP	1 CUP	215	55
APRICOT, CANNED, HEAVY SYRUP	3 HALVES	70	18

Food		Calories	Carbs
ARTICHOKES, GLOBE, COOKED, DRN	1 ARTCHK	55	12
ASPARAGUS, CKD FRM FRZ,DRN,CUT	1 CUP	50	9
ASPARAGUS, CKD FRM FRZ,DR,SPER	4 SPEARS	15	3
ASPARAGUS, CKD FRM RAW, DR,CUT	1 CUP	45	8
ASPARAGUS, CKD FRM RAW,DR,SPER	4 SPEARS	15	3
ASPARAGUS,CANNED,SPEARS,NOSALT	4 SPEARS	10	2
ASPARAGUS,CANNED,SPEARS,W/SALT	4 SPEARS	10	2
AVOCADOS, CALIFORNIA	1 AVOCADO	30	305
AVOCADOS, FLORIDA	1 AVOCDO	340	27
BAGELS, EGG	1 BAGEL	200	38
BAGELS, PLAIN	1 BAGEL	200	38
BAKING POWDER, LOW SODIUM	1 TSP	5	1
BAKING POWDER, STRGHT PHOSPHAT	1 TSP	5	1
BAKING POWDER,SAS, CA PO4	1 TSP	5	1
BAKING POWDER,SAS,CAPO4+CASO4	1 TSP	5	1
BAKING PWDR BISCUITS,FROM MIX	1 BISCUT	95	12
BAKING PWDR BISCUITS,HOMERECPE	1 BISCUT	100	13
BAKING PWDR BISCUITS,REFRGDOGH	1 BISCUT	65	10
BAMBOO SHOOTS, CANNED, DRAINED	1 CUP	25	4
BANANAS	1 BANANA	105	27
BANANAS, SLICED	1 CUP	140	35
BARBECUE SAUCE	1 TBSP	10	10
BARLEY, PEARLED,LIGHT, UNCOOKD	1 CUP	700	158
BEAN SPROUTS, MUNG, COOKD,DRAN	1 CUP	25	5
BEAN SPROUTS, MUNG, RAW	1 CUP	30	6
BEAN WITH BACON SOUP, CANNED	1 CUP	170	23
BEANS,DRY,CANNED,W/FRANKFURTER	1 CUP	365	32
BEANS,DRY,CANNED,W/PORK+SWTSCE	1 CUP	385	54
BEANS,DRY,CANNED,W/PORK+TOMSCE	1 CUP	310	48

Food		Calories	Carbs
BEEF AND VEGETABLE STEW,HM RCP	1 CUP	220	15
BEEF BROTH, BOULLN, CONSM,CNND	1 CUP	15	0
BEEF GRAVY, CANNED	1 CUP	125	11
BEEF HEART, BRAISED	3 OZ	150	0
BEEF LIVER, FRIED	3 OZ	185	7
BEEF NOODLE SOUP, CANNED	1 CUP	85	9
BEEF POTPIE, HOME RECIPE	1 PIECE	515	39
BEEF ROAST, EYE O RND, LEAN2.	6 OZ	135	0
BEEF ROAST, EYE O RND,LEAN+FAT	3 OZ	205	0
BEEF ROAST, RIB, LEAN ONLY	2.2 OZ	150	0
BEEF ROAST, RIB, LEAN + FAT	3 OZ	315	0
BEEF STEAK,SIRLOIN,BROIL,LEAN	2.5 OZ	150	0
BEEF STEAK,SIRLOIN,BROIL,LN+FT	3 OZ	240	0
BEEF, CANNED, CORNED	3 OZ	185	0
BEEF, CKD,BTTM ROUND,LEAN ONLY	2.8 OZ	175	0
BEEF, CKD,BTTM ROUND,LEAN+ FAT	3 OZ	220	0
BEEF, CKD,CHUCK BLADE,LEANONLY	2.2 OZ	170	0
BEEF, CKD,CHUCK BLADE,LEAN+FAT	3 OZ	325	0
BEEF, DRIED, CHIPPED	2.5 OZ	145	0
BEER, LIGHT	12 FL OZ	95	5
BEER, REGULAR	12 FL OZ	150	13
BEET GREENS, COOKED, DRAINED	1 CUP	40	8
BEETS, CANNED, DRAINED,NO SALT	1 CUP	55	12
BEETS, CANNED, DRAINED,W/ SALT	1 CUP	55	12
BEETS, COOKED, DRAINED, DICED	1 CUP	55	11
BEETS, COOKED, DRAINED, WHOLE	2 BEETS	30	7
BLACK-EYED PEAS, DRY, COOKED	1 CUP	190	35
BLACK BEANS, DRY, COOKED,DRAND	1 CUP	225	41
BLACKBERRIES, RAW	1 CUP	75	18

Food		Calories	Carbs
BLACKEYE PEAS, IMMATR,RAW,CKED	1 CUP	180	30
BLACKEYE PEAS,IMMTR,FRZN,CKED	1 CUP	225	40
BLUE CHEESE	1 OZ	100	1
BLUE CHEESE SALAD DRESSING	1 TBSP	8	75
BLUEBERRIES, FROZEN, SWEETENED	1 CUP	185	50
BLUEBERRIES, FROZEN, SWEETENED	10 OZ	230	62
BLUEBERRIES, RAW	1 CUP	80	20
BLUEBERRY MUFFINS, HOME RECIPE	1 MUFFIN	135	20
BLUEBERRY MUFFINS,FROM COM MIX	1 MUFFIN	140	22
BLUEBERRY PIE	1 PIE	2285	330
BLUEBERRY PIE	1 PIECE	380	55
BOLOGNA	2 SLICES	180	2
BOSTON BROWN BREAD,W/WHTECRNM	1 SLICE	95	21
BOSTON BROWN BREAD,W/YLLWCRNML	1 SLICE	95	21
BOUILLON, DEHYDRTD, UNPREPARED	1 PKT	15	1
BRAN MUFFINS, FROM COMMERL MIX	1 MUFFIN	140	24
BRAN MUFFINS, HOME RECIPE	1 MUFFIN	125	19
BRAUNSCHWEIGER	2 SLICES	205	2
BRAZIL NUTS	1 OZ	185	4
BREAD STUFFING,FROM MX,DRYTYPE	1 CUP	500	50
BREAD STUFFING,FROM MX,MOIST	1 CUP	420	40
BREADCRUMBS, DRY, GRATED	1 CUP	390	73
BROCCOLI, FRZN, COOKED, DRANED	1 CUP	50	10
BROCCOLI, FRZN, COOKED, DRANED	1 PIECE	10	2
BROCCOLI, RAW	1 SPEAR	40	8
BROCCOLI, RAW, COOKED, DRAINED	1 CUP	9	5
BROCCOLI, RAW, COOKED, DRAINED	1 SPEAR	50	10
BROWN AND SERVE SAUSAGE,BRWND	1 LINK	50	0
BROWN GRAVY FROM DRY MIX	1 CUP	80	14

Food		Calories	Carbs
BROWNIES W/ NUTS,FRM HOME RECP	1 BROWNE	95	11
BROWNIES W/ NUTS,FRSTNG,CMMRCL	1 BROWNE	100	16
BRUSSELS SPROUTS, FRZN, COOKED	1 CUP	65	13
BRUSSELS SPROUTS, RAW, COOKED	1 CUP	60	13
BUCKWHEAT FLOUR, LIGHT, SIFTED	1 CUP	340	78
BULGUR, UNCOOKED	1 CUP	600	129
BUTTERMILK, DRIED	1 CUP	465	59
BUTTERMILK, FLUID	1 CUP	100	12
BUTTER, SALTED	1 PAT	35	0
BUTTER, SALTED	1 TBSP	100	0
BUTTER, SALTED	1/2 CUP	810	0
BUTTER, UNSALTED	1 PAT	35	0
BUTTER, UNSALTED	1 TBSP	100	0
BUTTER, UNSALTED	1/2 CUP	810	0
CABBAGE, CHINESE, PAK-CHOI,CKD	1 CUP	20	3
CABBAGE, CHINESE,PE-TSAI, RAW	1 CUP	10	2
CABBAGE, COMMON, COOKED, DRNED	1 CUP	30	7
CABBAGE, COMMON, RAW	1 CUP	15	4
CABBAGE, RED, RAW	1 CUP	20	4
CABBAGE, SAVOY, RAW	1 CUP	20	4
CAKE OR PASTRY FLOUR, SIFTED	1 CUP	350	76
CAMEMBERT CHEESE	1 WEDGE	115	0
CANTALOUP, RAW	1/2 MELN	95	22
CAP'N CRUNCH CEREAL	1 OZ	120	23
CARAMELS, PLAIN OR CHOCOLATE	1 OZ	115	22
CAROB FLOUR	1 CUP	255	126
CARROT CAKE,CREMCHESE FRST,REC	1 CAKE	6175	775
CARROT CAKE,CREAM CHESE FRST,REC	1 PIECE	385	48
CARROTS, CANNED, DRN, W/ SALT	1 CUP	35	8

Food		Calories	Carbs
CARROTS, COOKED FROM FROZEN	1 CUP	55	12
CARROTS, COOKED FROM RAW	1 CUP	70	16
CARROTS, RAW, GRATED	1 CUP	45	11
CARROTS, RAW, WHOLE	1 CARROT	30	7
CASHEW NUTS, DRY ROASTD,SALTED	1 OZ	165	9
CASHEW NUTS, DRY ROASTD,UNSALT	1 CUP	785	45
CASHEW NUTS, OIL ROASTD,UNSALT	1 CUP	750	37
CASHEW NUTS, OIL ROASTD,UNSALT	1 OZ	165	8
CATSUP	1 CUP	290	69
CATSUP	1 TBSP	15	4
CAULIFLOWER, COOKED FROM FROZN	1 CUP	35	7
CAULIFLOWER, COOKED FROM RAW	1 CUP	30	6
CAULIFLOWER, RAW	1 CUP	25	5
CELERY SEED	1 TSP	10	1
CELERY, PASCAL TYPE, RAW,PIECE	1 CUP	20	4
CELERY, PASCAL TYPE, RAW,STALK	1 STALK	5	1
CHEDDAR CHEESE	1 CU IN	70	0
CHEDDAR CHEESE	1 OZ	115	0
CHEDDDAR CHEESE, SHREDDED	1 CUP	455	1
CHEERIOS CEREAL	1 OZ	20	4
CHEESE CRACKERS, PLAIN	10 CRACK	50	6
CHEESE CRACKERS, SANDWCH,PEANT	1 SANDWH	40	5
CHEESE SAUCE W/ MILK, FRM MIX	1 CUP	305	23
CHEESEBURGER, 4OZ PATTY	1 SANDWH	525	40
CHEESEBURGER, REGULAR	1 SANDWH	300	28
CHEESECAKE	1 CAKE	3350	317
CHEESECAKE	1 PIECE	280	26
CHERRIES, SOUR,RED,CANND,WATER	1 CUP	90	22
CHERRIES, SWEET, RAW	10 CHERY	50	11

Food		Calories	Carbs
CHERRY PIE	1 PIE	2465	363
CHERRY PIE	1 PIECE	410	61
CHESTNUTS, EUROPEAN, ROASTED	1 CUP	3	350
CHICKEN A LA KING, HOME RECIPE	1 CUP	470	12
CHICKEN AND NOODLES, HOME RECP	1 CUP	365	6
CHICKEN CHOW MEIN, CANNED	1 CUP	95	18
CHICKEN CHOW MEIN, HOME RECIPE	1 CUP	255	10
CHICKEN FRANKFURTER	1 FRANK	115	3
CHICKEN GRAVY FROM DRY MIX	1 CUP	85	14
CHICKEN GRAVY, CANNED	1 CUP	190	13
CHICKEN LIVER, COOKED	1 LIVER	30	0
CHICKEN NOODLE SOUP, CANNED	1 CUP	75	9
CHICKEN NOODLE SOUP,DEHYD,PRPD	1 PKT	40	6
CHICKEN POTPIE, HOME RECIPE	1 PIECE	545	42
CHICKEN RICE SOUP, CANNED	1 CUP	60	7
CHICKEN ROLL, LIGHT	2 SLICES	90	1
CHICKEN, CANNED, BONELESS	5 OZ	235	0
CHICKEN, FRIED, BATTER, BREAST	4.9 OZ	365	13
CHICKEN, FRIED, BATTER,DRMSTCK	2.5 OZ	195	6
CHICKEN, FRIED, FLOUR, BREAST	3.5 OZ	220	2
CHICKEN, FRIED, FLOUR, DRMSTCK	1.7 OZ	120	1
CHICKEN, ROASTED, BREAST	3.0 OZ	140	0
CHICKEN, ROASTED, DRUMSTICK	1.6 OZ	75	0
CHICKEN, STEWED, LIGHT + DARK	1 CUP	250	0
CHICKPEAS, COOKED, DRAINED	1 CUP	270	45
CHILI CON CARNE W/ BEANS, CNND	1 CUP	340	31
CHILI POWDER	1 TSP	10	1
CHOCOLATE CHIP COOKIES,COMMRCL	4 COOKIE	180	28
CHOCOLATE CHIP COOKIES,HME RCP	4 COOKIE	185	26

Food		Calories	Carbs
CHOCOLATE CHIP COOKIES,REFRIG	4 COOKIE	225	32
CHOCOLATE MILK, LOWFAT 1%	1 CUP	160	26
CHOCOLATE MILK, LOWFAT 2%	1 CUP	180	26
CHOCOLATE MILK, REGULAR	1 CUP	210	26
CHOCOLATE, BITTER OT BAKING	1 OZ	145	8
CHOP SUEY W/ BEEF + PORK,HMRCP	1 CUP	300	13
CINNAMON	1 TSP	5	2
CLAM CHOWDER, MANHATTAN, CANND	1 CUP	80	12
CLAM CHOWDER, NEW ENG, W/ MILK	1 CUP	165	17
CLAMS, CANNED, DRAINED	3 OZ	85	2
CLAMS, RAW	3 OZ	65	2
CLUB SODA	12 FL OZ	0	0
COCOA PWDR W/O NOFAT DRYMLK,PRD	1 SERVNG	225	30
COCOA PWDR W/O NONFAT DRY MILK	3/4 OZ	75	19
COCOA PWDR WITH NONFAT DRYMILK	1 OZ	100	22
COCOA PWDR W/ NOFAT DRMLK,PRPD	1 SERVNG	100	22
COCONUT, DRIED, SWEETND,SHREDD	1 CUP	470	44
COCONUT, RAW, PIECE	1 PIECE	160	7
COCONUT, RAW, SHREDDED	1 CUP	285	12
COFFEECAKE, CRUMB, FROM MIX	1 CAKE	1385	225
COFFEECAKE, CRUMB, FROM MIX	1 PIECE	230	38
COFFEE, BREWED	6 FL OZ	0	0
COFFEE, INSTANT, PREPARED	6 FL OZ	0	1
COLA, DIET, ASPARTAME ONLY	12 FL OZ	0	0
COLA, DIET, ASPRTAME + SACCHRN	12 FL OZ	0	0
COLA, DIET, SACCHARIN ONLY	12 FL OZ	0	0
COLA, REGULAR	12 FL OZ	160	41
COLLARDS, COOKED FROM FROZEN	1 CUP	60	12
COLLARDS, COOKED FROM RAW	1 CUP	25	5

Food		Calories	Carbs
COOKED SALAD DRSSING, HOME RCP	1 TBSP	25	2
CORN CHIPS	1 OZ	155	16
CORN FLAKES, KELLOGG'S	1 OZ	110	24
CORN FLAKES, TOASTIES	1 OZ	110	24
CORN GRITS, COOKED, INSTANT	1 PKT	80	18
CORN GRITS,CKD,REG,WHTE,NOSALT	1 CUP	145	31
CORN GRITS,CKD,REG,WHTE,W/SALT	1 CUP	145	31
CORN GRITS,CKD,REG,YLLW,NOSALT	1 CUP	145	31
CORN GRITS,CKD,REG,YLLW,W/SALT	1 CUP	145	31
CORN MUFFINS, FROM COMMERL MIX	1 MUFFIN	145	22
CORN MUFFINS, HOME RECIPE	1 MUFFIN	145	21
CORN OIL	1 CUP	1925	0
CORN OIL	1 TBSP	125	0
CORNMEAL,BOLTED,DRY FORM	1 CUP	440	91
CORNMEAL,DEGERMED,ENRCHED,COOK	1 CUP	120	26
CORNMEAL,DEGERMED,ENRICHED,DRY	1 CUP	500	108
CORNMEAL,WHOLE-GRND,UNBOLT,DRY	1 CUP	435	90
CORN, CNND,CRM STL,WHIT,NO SAL	1 CUP	185	46
CORN, CNND,CRM STL,WHIT,W/SALT	1 CUP	185	46
CORN, CNND,CRM STL,YLLW,NO SAL	1 CUP	185	46
CORN, CNND,CRM STL,YLLW,W/SALT	1 CUP	185	46
CORN, COOKED FRM FROZN, WHITE	1 CUP	135	34
CORN, COOKED FRM FROZN, WHITE	1 EAR	60	14
CORN, COOKED FRM FROZN, YELLOW	1 CUP	135	34
CORN, COOKED FRM FROZN, YELLOW	1 EAR	60	14
CORN, COOKED FROM RAW, WHITE	1 EAR	85	19
CORN, COOKED FROM RAW, YELLOW	1 EAR	85	19
CORN,CNND,WHL KRNL,WHTE,NO SALT	1 CUP	165	41
CORN,CNND,WHL KRNL,WHTE,W/SALT	1 CUP	165	41

Food		Calories	Carbs
CORN,CNND,WHL KRNL,YLLW,NO SALT	1 CUP	165	41
CORN,CNND,WHL KRNL,YLLW,W/SALT	1 CUP	165	41
COTTAGE CHEESE,CREMD,LRGE CURD	1 CUP	235	6
COTTAGE CHEESE,CREMD,SMLL CURD	1 CUP	215	6
COTTAGE CHEESE,CREMD,W/FRUIT	1 CUP	280	30
COTTAGE CHEESE,LOWFAT 2%	1 CUP	205	8
COTTAGE CHEESE,UNCREAMED	1 CUP	125	3
CR OF CHICKEN SOUP W/ H20,CNND	1 CUP	115	9
CR OF CHICKEN SOUP W/ MLK,CNND	1 CUP	190	15
CR OF MUSHROM SOUP W/ H2O,CNND	1 CUP	130	9
CR OF MUSHROM SOUP W/ MLK,CNND	1 CUP	205	15
CRABMEAT, CANNED	1 CUP	135	1
CRACKED-WHEAT BREAD	1 LOAF	1190	227
CRACKED-WHEAT BREAD	1 SLICE	65	12
CRACKED-WHEAT BREAD, TOASTED	1 SLICE	65	12
CRANBERRY JUICE COCKTAL W/VITC	1 CUP	145	38
CRANBERRY SAUCE, CANNED,SWTND	1 CUP	420	108
CREAM CHEESE	1 OZ	100	1
CREAM OF WHEAT,CKD,MIX N EAT	1 PKT	100	21
CREME PIE	1 PIE	2710	351
CREME PIE	1 PIECE	455	59
CRM WHEAT,CKD, QUICK, NO SALT	1 CUP	140	29
CRM WHEAT,CKD,QUICK, W/ SALT	1 CUP	140	29
CRM WHEAT,CKD,REG,INST,NO SALT	1 CUP	140	29
CRM WHEAT,CKD,REG,INST,W/SALT	1 CUP	140	29
CROISSANTS	1 CROSST	235	27
CUCUMBER, W/ PEEL	6 SLICES	5	1
CURRY POWDER	1 TSP	5	1
CUSTARD PIE	1 PIE	1985	213

Food		Calories	Carbs
CUSTARD PIE	1 PIECE	330	36
CUSTARD, BAKED	1 CUP	305	29
DANDELION GREENS, COOKED, DRND	1 CUP	35	7
DANISH PASTRY, FRUIT	1 PASTRY	235	28
DANISH PASTRY, PLAIN, NO NUTS	1 OZ	110	13
DANISH PASTRY, PLAIN, NO NUTS	1 PASTRY	220	26
DANISH PASTRY, PLAIN, NO NUTS	1 RING	1305	152
DATES	10 DATES	230	61
DATES, CHOPPED	1 CUP	490	131
DEVIL'S FOOD CAKE,CHOCFRST,FMX	1 CAKE	3755	645
DEVIL'S FOOD CAKE,CHOCFRST,FMX	1 CUPCAK	120	20
DEVIL'S FOOD CAKE,CHOCFRST,FMX	1 PIECE	235	40
DOUGHNUTS, CAKE TYPE, PLAIN	1 DONUT	210	24
DOUGHNUTS, YEAST-LEAVEND,GLZED	1 DONUT	235	26
DUCK, ROASTED, FLESH ONLY	1/2 DUCK	445	0
EGGNOG	1 CUP	340	34
EGGPLANT, COOKED, STEAMED	1 CUP	25	6
EGGS, COOKED, FRIED	1 EGG	90	1
EGGS, COOKED, HARD-COOKED	1 EGG	75	1
EGGS, COOKED, POACHED	1 EGG	75	1
EGGS, COOKED, SCRAMBLED/OMELET	1 EGG	100	1
EGGS, RAW, WHITE	1 WHITE	15	0
EGGS, RAW, WHOLE	1 EGG	75	1
EGGS, RAW, YOLK	1 YOLK	60	0
ENCHILADA	1 ENCHLD	235	24
ENDIVE, CURLY, RAW	1 CUP	10	2
ENG MUFFIN, EGG, CHEESE, BACON	1 SANDWH	360	31
ENGLISH MUFFINS, PLAIN	1 MUFFIN	140	27
ENGLISH MUFFINS, PLAIN, TOASTD	1 MUFFIN	140	27

Food		Calories	Carbs
EVAPORATED MILK, SKIM, CANNED	1 CUP	200	29
EVAPORATED MILK, WHOLE, CANNED	1 CUP	340	25
FATS, COOKING/VEGETBL SHORTENG	1 CUP	1810	0
FATS, COOKING/VEGETBL SHORTENG	1 TBSP	115	0
FETA CHEESE	1 OZ	75	1
FIG BARS	4 COOKIE	210	42
FIGS, DRIED	10 FIGS	475	122
FILBERTS, (HAZELNUTS) CHOPPED	1 CUP	725	18
FILBERTS, (HAZELNUTS) CHOPPED	1 OZ	180	4
FISH SANDWICH, LGE, W/O CHEESE	1 SANDWH	470	41
FISH SANDWICH, REG, W/ CHEESE	1 SANDWH	420	39
FISH STICKS, FROZEN, REHEATED	1 STICK	70	4
FLOUNDER OR SOLE, BAKED, BUTTR	3 OZ	120	0
FLOUNDER OR SOLE, BAKED,MARGRN	3 OZ	6	120
FLOUNDER OR SOLE, BAKED,W/OFAT	3 OZ	80	0
FONDANT, UNCOATED	1 OZ	105	27
FRANKFURTER, COOKED	1 FRANK	145	1
FRENCH BREAD	1 SLICE	100	18
FRENCH OR VIENNA BREAD	1 LOAF	1270	230
FRENCH SALAD DRESSING, LOCALOR	1 TBSP	25	2
FRENCH SALAD DRESSING, REGULAR	1 TBSP	85	1
FRENCH TOAST, HOME RECIPE	1 SLICE	155	17
FRIED PIE, APPLE	1 PIE	255	31
FRIED PIE, CHERRY	1 PIE	250	32
FROOT LOOPS CEREAL	1 OZ	110	25
FRUIT COCKTAIL,CNND,HEAVYSYRUP	1 CUP	185	48
FRUIT COCKTAIL,CNND,JUICE PACK	1 CUP	115	29
FRUIT PUNCH DRINK, CANNED	6 FL OZ	85	22
FRUITCAKE,DARK, FROM HOMERECIP	1 CAKE	783	74

Food		Calories	Carbs
FRUITCAKE,DARK, FROM HOMERECIP	1 PIECE	165	25
FUDGE, CHOCOLATE, PLAIN	1 OZ	115	21
GARLIC POWDER	1 TSP	10	2
GELATIN DESSERT, PREPARED	1/2 CUP	70	17
GELATIN, DRY	1 ENVELP	25	0
GINGER ALE	12 FL OZ	125	32
GINGERBREAD CAKE, FROM MIX	1 CAKE	1575	291
GINGERBREAD CAKE, FROM MIX	1 PIECE	175	32
GIN,RUM,VODKA,WHISKY 80-PROOF	1.5 F OZ	95	0
GIN,RUM,VODKA,WHISKY 86-PROOF	1.5 F OZ	105	0
GIN,RUM,VODKA,WHISKY 90-PROOF	1.5 F OZ	110	0
GOLDEN GRAHAMS CEREAL	1 OZ	110	24
GRAHAM CRACKER, PLAIN	2 CRACKR	60	11
GRAPE-NUTS CEREAL	1 OZ	100	23
GRAPE DRINK, CANNED	6 FL OZ	100	26
GRAPE JUICE, CANNED	1 CUP	155	38
GRAPE SODA	12 FL OZ	180	46
GRAPEFRT JCE,FRZN,CNCN,UNSWTEN	6 FL OZ	300	72
GRAPEFRT JCE,FRZN,DLTD,UNSWTEN	1 CUP	100	24
GRAPEFRUIT JUICE, CANNED,SWTND	1 CUP	115	28
GRAPEFRUIT JUICE, CANNED,UNSWT	1 CUP	95	22
GRAPEFRUIT JUICE, RAW	1 CUP	95	23
GRAPEFRUIT, CANNED, SYRUP PACK	1 CUP	150	39
GRAPEFRUIT, RAW, PINK	1/2 FRUT	40	10
GRAPEFRUIT, RAW, WHITE	1/2 FRUT	40	10
GRAPEJCE,FRZN,CONCEN,SWTND,W/C	6 FL OZ	385	96
GRAPEJCE,FRZN,DILUTD,SWTND,W/C	1 CUP	125	32
GRAPES, EUROPEAN, RAW, THOMPSN	10 GRAPE	35	9
GRAPES, EUROPEAN, RAW, TOKAY	10 GRAPE	40	10

Food		Calories	Carbs
GRAVY AND TURKEY, FROZEN	5 OZ	95	7
GREAT NORTHN BEANS,DRY,CKD,DRN	1 CUP	210	38
GROUND BEEF, BROILED, LEAN	3 OZ	230	0
GROUND BEEF, BROILED, REGULAR	3 OZ	245	0
GUM DROPS	1 OZ	100	25
HADDOCK, BREADED, FRIED	3 OZ	175	7
HALF AND HALF, CREAM	1 CUP	315	10
HALF AND HALF, CREAM	1 TBSP	20	1
HALIBUT, BROILED, BUTTER,LEMJU	3 OZ	140	0
HAMBURGER, 4OZ PATTY	1 SANDWH	445	38
HAMBURGER, REGULAR	1 SANDWH	245	28
HARD CANDY	1 OZ	110	28
HERRING, PICKLED	3 OZ	190	0
HOLLANDAISE SCE, W/ H2O,FRM MX	1 CUP	240	14
HONEY	1 CUP	1030	279
HONEY	1 TBSP	65	17
HONEY NUT CHEERIOS CEREAL	1 OZ	105	23
HONEYDEW MELON, RAW	1/10 MEL	45	12
ICE CREAM, VANLLA, REGULR 11%	1 CUP	270	32
ICE CREAM, VANLLA, REGULR 11%	1/2 GALN	2155	254
ICE CREAM, VANLLA, REGULR 11%	3 FL OZ	100	12
ICE CREAM, VANLLA, RICH 16% FT	1 CUP	350	32
ICE CREAM, VANLLA, RICH 16% FT	1/2 GAL	2805	256
ICE CREAM, VANLLA, SOFT SERVE	1 CUP	375	38
ICE MILK, VANILLA, 4% FAT	1 CUP	185	29
ICE MILK, VANILLA, 4% FAT	1/2 GAL	1470	232
ICE MILK, VANILLA,SOFTSERV 3%	1 CUP	225	38
IMITATION CREAMERS, LIQUID FRZ	1 TBSP	20	2
IMITATION CREAMERS, POWDERED	1 TSP	10	1

Food		Calories	Carbs
IMITATION WHIPPED TOPPING,FRZN	1 CUP	240	17
IMITATION WHIPPED TOPPING,FRZN	1 TBSP	15	1
IMITATN SOUR DRESSING	1 CUP	415	11
IMITATN SOUR DRESSING	1 TBSP	20	1
IMITATN WHIPD TOPING,PRESSRZD	1 CUP	185	11
IMITATN WHIPD TOPING,PRESSRZD	1 TBSP	10	1
IMITATN WHIPD TOPING,PWDRD,PRP	1 CUP	150	13
IMITATN WHIPD TOPING,PWDRD,PRP	1 TBSP	10	1
ITALIAN BREAD	1 LOAF	1255	256
ITALIAN BREAD	1 SLICE	85	17
ITALIAN SALAD DRESSING,LOCALOR	1 TBSP	5	2
ITALIAN SALAD DRESSING,REGULAR	1 TBSP	80	1
JAMS AND PRESERVES	1 PKT	40	10
JAMS AND PRESERVES	1 TBSP	55	14
JELLIES	1 PKT	40	10
JELLIES	1 TBSP	50	13
JELLY BEANS	1 OZ	105	26
JERUSALEM-ARTICHOKE, RAW	1 CUP	115	26
KALE, COOKED FROM FROZEN	1 CUP	40	7
KALE, COOKED FROM RAW	1 CUP	40	7
KIWIFRUIT, RAW	1 KIWI	45	11
KOHLRABI, COOKED, DRAINED	1 CUP	50	11
LAMB, RIB, ROASTED, LEAN ONLY	2 OZ	130	0
LAMB, RIB, ROASTED, LEAN + FAT	3 OZ	315	0
LAMB,CHOPS,ARM,BRAISED,LEAN	1.7 OZ	135	0
LAMB,CHOPS,ARM,BRAISED,LEAN+FT	2.2 OZ	220	0
LAMB,CHOPS,LOIN,BROIL,LEAN	2.3 OZ	140	0
LAMB,CHOPS,LOIN,BROIL,LEAN+FAT	2.8 OZ	235	0
LAMB,LEG,ROASTED, LEAN ONLY	2.6 OZ	140	0

Food		Calories	Carbs
LAMB,LEG,ROASTED, LEAN+ FAT	3 OZ	205	0
LARD	1 CUP	1850	0
LARD	1 TBSP	115	0
LEMON-LIME SODA	12 FL OZ	155	39
LEMON JUICE, CANNED	1 CUP	50	16
LEMON JUICE, CANNED	1 TBSP	5	1
LEMON JUICE, RAW	1 CUP	60	21
LEMON JUICE,FRZN,SINGLE-STRNGH	6 FL OZ	55	16
LEMON MERINGUE PIE	1 PIE	2140	317
LEMON MERINGUE PIE	1 PIECE	355	53
LEMONADE,CONCENTRATE,FRZ,UNDIL	6 FL OZ	425	112
LEMONADE,CONCEN,FRZEN,DILUTED	6 FL OZ	80	21
LEMONS, RAW	1 LEMON	15	5
LENTILS, DRY, COOKED	1 CUP	215	38
LETTUCE, BUTTERHEAD, RAW,HEAD	1 HEAD	20	4
LETTUCE, BUTTERHEAD, RAW,LEAVE	1 LEAF	0	0
LETTUCE, CRISPHEAD, RAW, HEAD	1 HEAD	70	11
LETTUCE, CRISPHEAD, RAW,PIECES	1 CUP	5	1
LETTUCE, CRISPHEAD, RAW,WEDGE	1 WEDGE	20	3
LETTUCE, LOOSELEAF	1 CUP	10	2
LIGHT, COFFEE OR TABLE CREAM	1 CUP	470	9
LIGHT, COFFEE OR TABLE CREAM	1 TBSP	30	1
LIMA BEANS, DRY, COOKED,DRANED	1 CUP	260	49
LIMA BEANS,BABY, FRZN,CKED,DRN	1 CUP	190	35
LIMA BEANS,THICK SEED,FRZN,CKD	1 CUP	170	32
LIME JUICE, RAW	1 CUP	65	22
LIME JUICE,CANNED	1 CUP	50	16
LIMEADE,CONCENTRATE,FRZN,UNDIL	6 FL OZ	410	108
LIMEADE,CONCEN,FROZEN,DILUTED	6 FL OZ	75	20

Food		Calories	Carbs
LUCKY CHARMS CEREAL	1 OZ	110	23
MACADAMIA NUTS, OILRSTD,SALTED	1 CUP	960	17
MACADAMIA NUTS, OILRSTD,SALTED	1 OZ	205	4
MACADAMIA NUTS, OILRSTD,UNSALT	1 CUP	960	17
MACADAMIA NUTS, OILRSTD,UNSALT	1 OZ	205	4
MACARONI AND CHEESE, CANNED	1 CUP	230	26
MACARONI AND CHEESE, HOME RCPE	1 CUP	430	40
MACARONI, COOKED, FIRM	1 CUP	190	39
MACARONI, COOKED, TENDER, HOT	1 CUP	155	32
MACARONI, COOKED, TENDER,COLD	1 CUP	115	24
MALT-O-MEAL, WITH SALT	1 CUP	120	26
MALT-O-MEAL, W/O SALT	1 CUP	120	26
MALTED MILK, CHOCOLATE, POWDER	3/4 OZ	85	18
MALTED MILK,CHOCOLATE, PWDRPPD	1 SERVNG	235	29
MALTED MILK,NATURAL, POWDER	3/4 OZ	85	15
MALTED MILK,NATURAL, PWDR PPRD	1 SERVNG	235	27
MANGOS, RAW	1 MANGO	135	35
MARGARINE, IMITATION 40% FAT	1 TBSP	50	0
MARGARINE, IMITATION 40% FAT	8 OZ	785	1
MARGARINE, REGULR,HARD,80% FAT	1 PAT	35	0
MARGARINE, REGULR,HARD,80% FAT	1 TBSP	100	0
MARGARINE, REGULR,HARD,80% FAT	1/2 CUP	810	1
MARGARINE, REGULR,SOFT,80% FAT	1 TBSP	100	0
MARGARINE, REGULR,SOFT,80% FAT	8 OZ	1625	1
MARGARINE, SPREAD,HARD,60% FAT	1 PAT	25	0
MARGARINE, SPREAD,HARD,60% FAT	1 TBSP	75	0
MARGARINE, SPREAD,HARD,60% FAT	1/2 CUP	610	0
MARGARINE, SPREAD,SOFT,60% FAT	1 TBSP	75	0
MARGARINE, SPREAD,SOFT,60% FAT	8 OZ	1225	0

Food		Calories	Carbs
MARSHMALLOWS	1 OZ	90	23
MAYONNAISE TYPE SALAD DRESSING	1 TBSP	60	4
MAYONNAISE, IMITATION	1 TBSP	35	2
MAYONNAISE, REGULAR	1 TBSP	100	0
MELBA TOAST, PLAIN	1 PIECE	20	4
MILK CHOCOLATE CANDY, PLAIN	1 OZ	145	16
MILK CHOCOLATE CANDY,W/ ALMOND	1 OZ	150	15
MILK CHOCOLATE CANDY,W/ PENUTS	1 OZ	155	13
MILK CHOCOLATE CANDY,W/ RICE C	1 OZ	140	18
MILK, LOFAT, 1%, ADDED SOLIDS	1 CUP	105	12
MILK, LOFAT, 1%, NO ADDEDSOLID	1 CUP	100	12
MILK, LOFAT, 2%, ADDED SOLIDS	1 CUP	125	12
MILK, LOFAT, 2%, NO ADDEDSOLID	1 CUP	120	12
MILK, SKIM, ADDED MILK SOLIDS	1 CUP	90	12
MILK, SKIM, NO ADDED MILKSOLID	1 CUP	85	12
MILK, WHOLE, 3.3% FAT	1 CUP	150	11
MINESTRONE SOUP, CANNED	1 CUP	80	11
MISO	1 CUP	470	65
MIXED GRAIN BREAD	1 LOAF	1165	212
MIXED GRAIN BREAD	1 SLICE	65	12
MIXED GRAIN BREAD, TOASTED	1 SLICE	65	12
MIXED NUTS W/ PEANTS,DRY,SALTD	1 OZ	170	7
MIXED NUTS W/ PEANTS,DRY,UNSLT	1 OZ	170	7
MIXED NUTS W/ PEANTS,OIL,SALTD	1 OZ	175	6
MIXED NUTS W/ PEANTS,OIL,UNSLT	1 OZ	175	6
MOLASSES, CANE, BLACKSTRAP	2 TBSP	85	22
MOZZARELLA CHEESE, WHOLE MILK	1 OZ	80	1
MOZZARELLA CHESE,SKIM, LOMOIST	1 OZ	80	1
MUENSTER CHEESE	1 OZ	105	0

Food		Calories	Carbs
MUSHROOM GRAVY, CANNED	1 CUP	120	13
MUSHROOMS, CANNED, DRND,W/SALT	1 CUP	35	8
MUSHROOMS, COOKED, DRAINED	1 CUP	40	8
MUSHROOMS, RAW	1 CUP	20	3
MUSTARD GREENS, COOKED, DRANED	1 CUP	20	3
MUSTARD, PREPARED, YELLOW	1 TSP	5	0
NATURE VALLEY GRANOLA CEREAL	1 OZ	125	19
NECTARINES, RAW	1 NECTRN	65	16
NONFAT DRY MILK, INSTANTIZED	1 CUP	245	35
NONFAT DRY MILK, INSTANTIZED	1 ENVLPE	325	47
NOODLES, CHOW MEIN, CANNED	1 CUP	220	26
NOODLES, EGG, COOKED	1 CUP	200	37
OATMEAL BREAD	1 LOAF	1145	212
OATMEAL BREAD	1 SLICE	65	12
OATMEAL BREAD, TOASTED	1 SLICE	65	12
OATMEAL W/ RAISINS COOKIES	4 COOKIE	245	36
OATMEAL,CKD,INSTNT,FLVRD,FORTF	1 PKT	160	31
OATMEAL,CKD,INSTNT,PLAIN,FORTF	1 PKT	105	18
OATMEAL,CKD,RG,QCK,INST,W/OSAL	1 CUP	145	25
OATMEAL,CKD,RG,QCK,INST,W/SALT	1 CUP	145	25
OCEAN PERCH, BREADED, FRIED	1 FILLET	185	7
OKRA PODS, COOKED	8 PODS	25	6
OLIVE OIL	1 CUP	1910	0
OLIVE OIL	1 TBSP	125	0
OLIVES, CANNED, GREEN	4 MEDIUM	15	0
OLIVES, CANNED, RIPE, MISSION	3 SMALL	15	0
ONION POWDER	1 TSP	5	2
ONION RINGS, BREADED,FRZN,PRPD	2 RINGS	80	8
ONION SOUP, DEHYDRATD, PREPRED	1 PKT	20	4

Food		Calories	Carbs
ONION SOUP, DEHYDRTD, UNPRPRED	1 PKT	20	4
ONIONS, RAW, CHOPPED	1 CUP	55	12
ONIONS, RAW, COOKED, DRAINED	1 CUP	60	13
ONIONS, RAW, SLICED	1 CUP	40	8
ONIONS, SPRING, RAW	6 ONION	10	2
ORANGE JUICE, CANNED	1 CUP	105	25
ORANGE JUICE, CHILLED	1 CUP	110	25
ORANGE JUICE, RAW	1 CUP	110	27
ORANGE SODA	12 FL OZ	180	46
ORANGE + GRAPEFRUIT JUCE,CANND	1 CUP	105	25
ORANGES, RAW	1 ORANGE	60	15
ORANGES, RAW, SECTIONS	1 CUP	85	21
OREGANO	1 TSP	5	1
OYSTERS, BREADED, FRIED	1 OYSTER	90	5
OYSTERS, RAW	1 CUP	160	8
PANCAKES, BUCKWHEAT, FROM MIX	1 PANCAK	55	6
PANCAKES, PLAIN, FROM MIX	1 PANCAK	60	8
PANCAKES, PLAIN, HOME RECIPE	1 PANCAK	60	9
PAPAYAS, RAW	1 CUP	65	17
PAPRIKA	1 TSP	5	1
PARMESAN CHEESE, GRATED	1 CUP	455	4
PARMESAN CHEESE, GRATED	1 OZ	130	1
PARMESAN CHEESE, GRATED	1 TBSP	25	0
PARSLEY, FREEZE-DRIED	1 TBSP	0	0
PARSLEY, RAW	10 SPRIG	5	1
PARSNIPS, COOKED, DRAINED	1 CUP	125	30
PASTERZD PROCES CHEESE, SWISS	1 OZ	95	1
PASTERZD PROCES CHEESE,AMERICN	1 OZ	105	0
PASTERZD PROCES CHESE FOOD,AMR	1 OZ	95	2

Food		Calories	Carbs
PASTERZD PROCES CHESE SPRED,AM	1 OZ	80	2
PEA BEANS, DRY, COOKED,DRAINED	1 CUP	225	40
PEACH PIE	1 PIE	2410	361
PEACH PIE	1 PIECE	405	60
PEACHES, CANNED, HEAVY SYRUP	1 CUP	190	51
PEACHES, CANNED, HEAVY SYRUP	1 HALF	60	16
PEACHES, CANNED, JUICE PACK	1 CUP	110	29
PEACHES, CANNED, JUICE PACK	1 HALF	35	9
PEACHES, DRIED	1 CUP	380	98
PEACHES, DRIED,COOKED,UNSWETND	1 CUP	200	51
PEACHES, FROZEN,SWETNED,W/VITC	1 CUP	235	60
PEACHES, FROZEN,SWETNED,W/VITC	10 OZ	265	68
PEACHES, RAW	1 PEACH	35	10
PEACHES, RAW, SLICED	1 CUP	75	19
PEANUT BUTTER	1 TBSP	95	3
PEANUT BUTTER COOKIE,HOME RECP	4 COOKIE	245	28
PEANUT OIL	1 CUP	1910	0
PEANUT OIL	1 TBSP	125	0
PEANUTS, OIL ROASTED, SALTED	1 CUP	840	27
PEANUTS, OIL ROASTED, SALTED	1 OZ	165	5
PEANUTS, OIL ROASTED, UNSALTED	1 CUP	840	27
PEANUTS, OIL ROASTED, UNSALTED	1 OZ	165	5
PEARS, CANNED, HEAVY SYRUP	1 CUP	190	49
PEARS, CANNED, HEAVY SYRUP	1 HALF	60	15
PEARS, CANNED, JUICE PACK	1 CUP	125	32
PEARS, CANNED, JUICE PACK	1 HALF	40	10
PEARS, RAW, BARTLETT	1 PEAR	100	25
PEARS, RAW, BOSC	1 PEAR	85	21
PEARS, RAW, D'ANJOU	1 PEAR	120	30

Food		Calories	Carbs
PEAS, EDIBLE POD, COOKED,DRNED	1 CUP	65	11
PEAS, GREEN,CNND,DRND, W/ SALT	1 CUP	115	21
PEAS, GREEN,CNND,DRND,W/O SALT	1 CUP	115	21
PEAS, SPLIT, DRY, COOKED	1 CUP	230	42
PEAS,GRN, FROZEN COOKED,DRANED	1 CUP	125	23
PEA, GREEN, SOUP, CANNED	1 CUP	165	27
PECAN PIE	1 PIE	3450	423
PECAN PIE	1 PIECE	575	71
PECANS, HALVES	1 CUP	720	20
PECANS, HALVES	1 OZ	190	5
PEPPER-TYPE SODA	12 FL OZ	160	41
PEPPERS, HOT CHILI, RAW, GREEN	1 PEPPER	20	4
PEPPERS, HOT CHILI, RAW, RED	1 PEPPER	20	4
PEPPERS, SWEET, COOKED, GREEN	1 PEPPER	15	3
PEPPERS, SWEET, COOKED, RED	1 PEPPER	15	3
PEPPERS, SWEET, RAW, GREEN	1 PEPPER	20	4
PEPPERS, SWEET, RAW, RED	1 PEPPER	20	4
PEPPER, BLACK	1 TSP	5	1
PICKLES, CUCUMBER, DILL	1 PICKLE	5	1
PICKLES, CUCUMBER, FRESH PACK	2 SLICES	10	3
PICKLES, CUCUMBER, SWT GHERKIN	1 PICKLE	20	5
PIECRUST, FROM MIX	2 CRUST	1485	141
PIECRUST,FROM HOME RECIPE	1 SHELL	900	79
PINE NUTS	1 OZ	160	5
PINEAPPLE-GRAPEFRUIT JUICEDRNK	6 FL OZ	90	23
PINEAPPLE JUICE, CANNED,UNSWTN	1 CUP	140	34
PINEAPPLE, CANNED, HEAVY SYRUP	1 CUP	200	52
PINEAPPLE, CANNED, HEAVY SYRUP	1 SLICE	45	12
PINEAPPLE, CANNED, JUICE PACK	1 CUP	150	39

Food		Calories	Carbs
PINEAPPLE, CANNED, JUICE PACK	1 SLICE	35	9
PINEAPPLE, RAW, DICED	1 CUP	75	19
PINTO BEANS,DRY,COOKED,DRAINED	1 CUP	265	49
PISTACHIO NUTS	1 OZ	165	7
PITA BREAD	1 PITA	165	33
PIZZA, CHEESE	1 SLICE	290	39
PLANTAINS, COOKED	1 CUP	180	48
PLANTAINS, RAW	1 PLANTN	220	57
PLUMS, CANNED, HEAVY SYRUP	1 CUP	230	60
PLUMS, CANNED, HEAVY SYRUP	3 PLUMS	120	31
PLUMS, CANNED, JUICE PACK	1 CUP	145	38
PLUMS, CANNED, JUICE PACK	3 PLUMS	55	14
PLUMS, RAW, 1-1/2-IN DIAM	1 PLUM	15	4
PLUMS, RAW, 2-1/8-IN DIAM	1 PLUM	35	9
POPCORN, AIR-POPPED, UNSALTED	1 CUP	30	6
POPCORN, POPPED, VEG OIL,SALTD	1 CUP	55	6
POPCORN, SUGAR SYRUP COATED	1 CUP	135	30
POPSICLE	1 POPCLE	70	18
PORK CHOP, LOIN, BROIL, LEAN	2.5 OZ	165	0
PORK CHOP, LOIN, BROIL, LEN+FT	3.1 OZ	275	0
PORK CHOP, LOIN,PANFRY, LEAN	2.4 OZ	180	0
PORK CHOP, LOIN,PANFRY,LEAN+FT	3.1 OZ	335	0
PORK FRESH HAM, ROASTD, LEAN	2.5 OZ	160	0
PORK FRESH HAM, ROASTD,LEAN+FT	3 OZ	250	0
PORK FRESH RIB, ROASTD, LEAN	2.5 OZ	175	0
PORK FRESH RIB, ROASTD,LEAN+FT	3 OZ	270	0
PORK SHOULDER, BRAISD, LEAN	2.4 OZ	165	0
PORK SHOULDER, BRAISD,LEAN+FAT	3 OZ	295	0
PORK, CURED, BACON, REGUL,CKED	3 SLICE	110	0

Food		Calories	Carbs
PORK, CURED, BACON,CANADN,CKED	2 SLICE	85	1
PORK, CURED, HAM, CANNED,ROAST	3 OZ	140	0
PORK, CURED, HAM, ROSTED,LEAN	2.4 OZ	105	0
PORK, CURED, HAM, ROSTED,LN+FT	3 OZ	205	0
PORK, LINK, COOKED	1 LINK	50	0
PORK, LUNCHEON MEAT,CANNED	2 SLICES	140	1
PORK, LUNCHEON MEAT,CHOPPD HAM	2 SLICES	95	0
PORK, LUNCHEON MEAT,CKD HAM,LN	2 SLICES	75	1
PORK, LUNCHEON MEAT,CKD HAM,RG	2 SLICES	105	2
POTATO CHIPS	10 CHIPS	105	10
POTATO SALAD MADE W/ MAYONNAIS	1 CUP	360	28
POTATOES, AU GRATIN, FROM MIX	1 CUP	230	31
POTATOES, AU GRATIN, HOME RECP	1 CUP	325	28
POTATOES, BAKED FLESH ONLY	1 POTATO	145	34
POTATOES, BAKED WITH SKIN	1 POTATO	220	51
POTATOES, BOILED, PEELED AFTER	1 POTATO	120	27
POTATOES, BOILED, PEELED BEFOR	1 POTATO	115	27
POTATOES, HASHED BROWN,FR FRZN	1 CUP	340	44
POTATOES, MASHED,FRM DEHYDRTED	1 CUP	235	32
POTATOES, MASHED,RECPE,MLK+MAR	1 CUP	225	35
POTATOES, MASHED,RECPE,W/ MILK	1 CUP	160	37
POTATOES, SCALLOPED, FROM MIX	1 CUP	230	31
POTATOES, SCALLOPED, HOME RECP	1 CUP	210	26
POTATOES,FRENCH-FRD,FRZN,FRIED	10 STRIP	160	20
POTATOES,FRENCH-FRD,FRZN,OVEN	10 STRIP	110	17
POUND CAKE, COMMERCIAL	1 LOAF	1935	257
POUND CAKE, COMMERCIAL	1 SLICE	110	15
POUND CAKE, FROM HOME RECIPE	1 LOAF	2025	265
POUND CAKE, FROM HOME RECIPE	1 SLICE	120	15

Food		Calories	Carbs
PRETZELS, STICK	10 PRETZ	10	2
PRETZELS, TWISTED, DUTCH	1 PRETZ	65	3
PRETZELS, TWISTED, THIN	10 PRETZ	240	48
PRODUCT 19 CEREAL	1 OZ	110	24
PROVOLONE CHEESE	1 OZ	100	1
PRUNE JUICE, CANNED	1 CUP	180	45
PRUNES, DRIED	5 LARGE	115	31
PRUNES, DRIED, COOKED,UNSWTNED	1 CUP	225	60
PUDDING, CHOCOLATE,CANNED	5 OZ	205	30
PUDDING, CHOC, COOKED FROM MIX	1/2 CUP	150	25
PUDDING, CHOC, INSTANT, FR MIX	1/2 CUP	155	27
PUDDING, RICE, FROM MIX	1/2 CUP	155	27
PUDDING, TAPIOCA, CANNED	5 OZ	160	28
PUDDING, TAPIOCA, FROM MIX	1/2 CUP	145	25
PUDDING, VANILLA, CANNED	5 OZ	220	33
PUDDING, VNLLA,COOKED FROM MIX	1/2 CUP	145	25
PUDDING, VNLLA,INSTANT FRM MIX	1/2 CUP	150	27
PUMPERNICKEL BREAD	1 LOAF	1160	218
PUMPERNICKEL BREAD	1 SLICE	80	16
PUMPERNICKEL BREAD, TOASTED	1 SLICE	80	16
PUMPKIN AND SQUASH KERNELS	1 OZ	155	5
PUMPKIN PIE	1 PIE	1920	223
PUMPKIN PIE	1 PIECE	320	37
PUMPKIN, CANNED	1 CUP	85	20
PUMPKIN, COOKED FROM RAW	1 CUP	50	12
QUICHE LORRAINE	1 SLICE	600	29
RADISHES, RAW	4 RADISH	5	1
RAISIN BRAN, KELLOGG'S	1 OZ	90	21
RAISIN BRAN, POST	1 OZ	85	21

Food		Calories	Carbs
RAISIN BREAD	1 LOAF	1260	239
RAISIN BREAD	1 SLICE	65	13
RAISIN BREAD, TOASTED	1 SLICE	65	13
RAISINS	1 CUP	435	115
RAISINS	1 PACKET	40	11
RASPBERRIES, FROZEN, SWEETENED	1 CUP	255	65
RASPBERRIES, FROZEN, SWEETENED	10 OZ	295	74
RASPBERRIES, RAW	1 CUP	60	14
RED KIDNEY BEANS, DRY, CANNED	1 CUP	230	42
REFRIED BEANS, CANNED	1 CUP	295	51
RELISH, SWEET	1 TBSP	20	5
RHUBARB, COOKED, ADDED SUGAR	1 CUP	280	75
RICE KRISPIES CEREAL	1 OZ	110	25
RICE, BROWN, COOKED	1 CUP	230	50
RICE, WHITE, COOKED	1 CUP	225	50
RICE, WHITE, INSTANT, COOKED	1 CUP	180	40
RICE, WHITE, PARBOILED, COOKED	1 CUP	185	41
RICE, WHITE, PARBOILED, RAW	1 CUP	685	150
RICE, WHITE, RAW	1 CUP	670	149
RICOTTA CHEESE, PART SKIM MILK	1 CUP	340	13
RICOTTA CHEESE, WHOLE MILK	1 CUP	430	7
ROAST BEEF SANDWICH	1 SANDWH	345	34
ROLLS, DINNER, COMMERCIAL	1 ROLL	85	14
ROLLS, DINNER, HOME RECIPE	1 ROLL	120	20
ROLLS, FRANKFURTER + HAMBURGER	1 ROLL	115	20
ROLLS, HARD	1 ROLL	155	30
ROLLS, HOAGIE OR SUBMARINE	1 ROLL	400	72
ROOT BEER	12 FL OZ	165	42
RYE BREAD, LIGHT	1 LOAF	1190	218

Food		Calories	Carbs
RYE BREAD, LIGHT	1 SLICE	65	12
RYE BREAD, LIGHT, TOASTED	1 SLICE	65	12
RYE WAFERS, WHOLE-GRAIN	2 WAFERS	55	10
SAFFLOWER OIL	1 CUP	1925	0
SAFFLOWER OIL	1 TBSP	125	0
SALAMI, COOKED TYPE	2 SLICES	145	1
SALAMI, DRY TYPE	2 SLICES	85	1
SALMON, BAKED, RED	3 OZ	140	0
SALMON, CANNED, PINK, W/ BONES	3 OZ	120	0
SALMON, SMOKED	3 OZ	150	0
SALT	1 TSP	0	0
SALTINES	4 CRACKR	50	9
SANDWICH SPREAD, PORK, BEEF	1 TBSP	35	2
SANDWICH TYPE COOKIE	4 COOKIE	195	29
SARDINES, ATLNTC,CNNED,OIL,DRN	3 OZ	175	0
SAUERKRAUT, CANNED	1 CUP	45	10
SCALLOPS, BREADED, FRZN,REHEAT	6 SCALOP	195	10
SEAWEED, KELP, RAW	1 OZ	10	3
SEAWEED, SPIRULINA, DRIED	1 OZ	80	7
SELF-RISING FLOUR, UNSIFTED	1 CUP	440	93
SEMISWEET CHOCOLATE	1 CUP	860	97
SESAME SEEDS	1 TBSP	45	1
SHAKES, THICK, CHOCOLATE	10 OZ	335	60
SHAKES, THICK, VANILLA	10 OZ	315	50
SHEETCAKE W/O FRSTNG,HOMERECIP	1 CAKE	2830	434
SHEETCAKE,W/ WHFRSTNG,HOMERCIP	1 CAKE	4020	694
SHEETCAKE,W/ WHFRSTNG,HOMERCIP	1 PIECE	445	77
SHEETCAKE,W/O FRSTNG,HOMERECIP	1 PIECE	315	48
SHERBET, 2% FAT	1 CUP	270	59

Food		Calories	Carbs
SHERBET, 2% FAT	1/2 GAL	2160	469
SHORTBREAD COOKIE, COMMERCIAL	4 COOKIE	155	20
SHORTBREAD COOKIE, HOME RECIPE	2 COOKIE	145	17
SHREDDED WHEAT CEREAL	1 OZ	100	23
SHRIMP, CANNED, DRAINED	3 OZ	100	1
SHRIMP, FRENCH FRIED	3 OZ	200	11
SNACK CAKES,DEVILS FOOD,CREMFLSM CAKE		105	17
SNACK CAKES,SPONGE CREME FLLNGSM CAKE		155	27
SNACK TYPE CRACKERS	1 CRACKR	15	2
SNAP BEAN,CNND,DRND,GREEN,SALT	1 CUP	25	6
SNAP BEAN,CNND,DRND,GRN,NOSALT	1 CUP	25	6
SNAP BEAN,CNND,DRND,YLLW, SALT	1 CUP	25	6
SNAP BEAN,CNND,DRND,YLLW,NOSAL	1 CUP	25	6
SNAP BEAN,FRZ,CKD,DRND,GREEN	1 CUP	35	8
SNAP BEAN,FRZ,CKD,DRND,YELLOW	1 CUP	35	8
SNAP BEAN,RAW,CKD,DRND,GREEN	1 CUP	45	10
SNAP BEAN,RAW,CKD,DRND,YELLOW	1 CUP	45	10
SOUR CREAM	1 CUP	495	10
SOUR CREAM	1 TBSP	25	1
SOY SAUCE	1 TBSP	10	2
SOYBEAN-COTTONSEED OIL, HYDRGN	1 CUP	1925	0
SOYBEAN-COTTONSEED OIL, HYDRGN	1 TBSP	125	0
SOYBEAN OIL, HYDROGENATED	1 CUP	1925	0
SOYBEAN OIL, HYDROGENATED	1 TBSP	125	0
SOYBEANS, DRY, COOKED, DRAINED	1 CUP	235	19
SPAGHETTI, COOKED, FIRM	1 CUP	190	39
SPAGHETTI, COOKED, TENDER	1 CUP	155	32
SPAGHETTI, TOM SAUCE CHEES,CND	1 CUP	190	39
SPAGHETTI, TOM SAUCE CHEE,HMRP	1 CUP	260	37

Food		Calories	Carbs
SPAGHETTI,MEATBALLS,TOMSAC,CND	1 CUP	260	29
SPAGHETTI,MEATBALLS,TOMSA,HMRP	1 CUP	330	39
SPECIAL K CEREAL	1 OZ	110	21
SPINACH SOUFFLE	1 CUP	220	3
SPINACH, CANNED, DRND,W/ SALT	1 CUP	50	7
SPINACH, CANNED, DRND,W/O SALT	1 CUP	50	7
SPINACH, COOKED FR FRZEN, DRND	1 CUP	55	10
SPINACH, COOKED FROM RAW, DRND	1 CUP	40	7
SPINACH, RAW	1 CUP	10	2
SQUASH, SUMMER, COOKED, DRAIND	1 CUP	35	8
SQUASH, WINTER, BAKED	1 CUP	80	18
STRAWBERRIES, FROZEN, SWEETEND	1 CUP	245	66
STRAWBERRIES, FROZEN, SWEETEND	10 OZ	275	74
STRAWBERRIES, RAW	1 CUP	45	10
SUGAR COOKIE, FROM REFRIG DOGH	4 COOKIE	235	31
SUGAR FROSTED FLAKES, KELLOGG	1 OZ	110	26
SUGAR SMACKS CEREAL	1 OZ	105	25
SUGAR, BROWN, PRESSED DOWN	1 CUP	820	212
SUGAR, POWDERED, SIFTED	1 CUP	385	100
SUGAR, WHITE, GRANULATED	1 CUP	770	199
SUGAR, WHITE, GRANULATED	1 PKT	25	6
SUGAR, WHITE, GRANULATED	1 TBSP	45	12
SUNFLOWER OIL	1 CUP	1925	0
SUNFLOWER OIL	1 TBSP	125	0
SUNFLOWER SEEDS	1 OZ	160	5
SUPER SUGAR CRISP CEREAL	1 OZ	105	26
SWEET (DARK) CHOCOLATE	1 OZ	150	16
SWEETENED CONDENSED MILK CNND	1 CUP	980	166
SWEETPOTATOES, BAKED, PEELED	1 POTATO	115	28

Food		Calories	Carbs
SWEETPOTATOES, BOILED W/O PEEL	1 POTATO	160	37
SWEETPOTATOES, CANDIED	1 PIECE	145	29
SWEETPOTATOES, CANNED, MASHED	1 CUP	260	59
SWEETPOTATOES, CNNED, VAC PACK	1 PIECE	35	8
SWISS CHEESE	1 OZ	105	1
SYRUP, CHOCOLATE FLAVORED THIN	2 TBSP	85	22
SYRUP, CHOCOLATE FLVRED, FUDGE	2 TBSP	125	21
TABLE SYRUP (CORN AND MAPLE)	2 TBSP	122	32
TACO	1 TACO	195	15
TAHINI	1 TBSP	90	3
TANGERINE JUICE, CANNED,SWTNED	1 CUP	125	30
TANGERINES, CANNED, LIGHT SYRP	1 CUP	155	41
TANGERINES, RAW	1 TANGRN	35	9
TARTAR SAUCE	1 TBSP	75	1
TEA, BREWED	8 FL OZ	0	0
TEA, INSTANT,PREPRD,UNSWEETEND	8 FL OZ	0	1
TEA,INSTANT,PREPARD,SWEETENED	8 FL OZ	85	22
TOASTER PASTRIES	1 PASTRY	210	38
TOFU	1 PIECE	85	3
TOMATO JUICE, CANNED WITH SALT	1 CUP	40	10
TOMATO JUICE, CANNED W/O SALT	1 CUP	40	10
TOMATO PASTE, CANNED WITH SALT	1 CUP	220	49
TOMATO PASTE, CANNED W/O SALT	1 CUP	220	49
TOMATO PUREE, CANNED WITH SALT	1 CUP	105	25
TOMATO PUREE, CANNED W/O SALT	1 CUP	105	25
TOMATO SAUCE, CANNED WITH SALT	1 CUP	75	18
TOMATO SOUP WITH MILK, CANNED	1 CUP	160	22
TOMATO SOUP W/ WATER, CANNED	1 CUP	85	17
TOMATO VEG SOUP, DEHYD,PREPRED	1 PKT	40	8

Food		Calories	Carbs
TOMATOES, CANNED, S+L, W/ SALT	1 CUP	50	10
TOMATOES, CANNED, S+L, W/O SALT	1 CUP	50	10
TOMATOES, RAW	1 TOMATO	25	5
TORTILLAS, CORN	1 TORTLA	65	13
TOTAL CEREAL	1 OZ	100	22
TRIX CEREAL	1 OZ	110	25
TROUT, BROILED, W/ BUTTR,LEMJU	3 OZ	175	0
TUNA SALAD	1 CUP	375	19
TUNA, CANND, DRND,OIL,CHK,LGHT	3 OZ	165	0
TUNA, CANND, DRND,WATR, WHITE	3 OZ	135	0
TURKEY HAM, CURED TURKEY THIGH	2 SLICES	75	0
TURKEY LOAF, BREAST MEAT W/O C	2 SLICES	45	0
TURKEY LOAF, BREAST MEAT, W/ C	2 SLICES	45	0
TURKEY PATTIES, BRD,BATTD,FRID	1 PATTY	180	10
TURKEY ROAST, FRZN,LGHT+DRK,CK	3 OZ	130	3
TURKEY, ROASTED, DARK MEAT	4 PIECES	160	0
TURKEY, ROASTED, LIGHT MEAT	2 PIECES	135	0
TURKEY, ROASTED, LIGHT + DARK	1 CUP	240	0
TURKEY, ROASTED, LIGHT + DARK	3 PIECES	145	0
TURNIP GREENS, CKED FRM FROZEN	1 CUP	50	8
TURNIP GREENS, COOKED FROM RAW	1 CUP	30	6
TURNIPS, COOKED, DICED	1 CUP	30	8
VANILLA WAFERS	10 COOKE	185	9
VEAL CUTLET, MED FAT,BRSD,BRLD	3 OZ	185	0
VEAL RIB, MED FAT, ROASTED	3 OZ	230	0
VEGETABLE BEEF SOUP, CANNED	1 CUP	80	10
VEGETABLE JUICE COCKTAIL, CNND	1 CUP	45	11
VEGETABLES, MIXED, CANNED	1 CUP	75	15
VEGETABLES, MIXED, CKED FR FRZ	1 CUP	105	24

Food		Calories	Carbs
VEGETARIAN SOUP, CANNED	1 CUP	70	12
VIENNA BREAD	1 SLICE	70	13
VIENNA SAUSAGE	1 SAUSAG	45	0
VINEGAR AND OIL SALAD DRESSING	1 TBSP	70	0
VINEGAR, CIDER	1 TBSP	0	1
WAFFLES, FROM HOME RECIPE	1 WAFFLE	245	26
WAFFLES, FROM MIX	1 WAFFLE	205	27
WALNUTS, BLACK, CHOPPED	1 CUP	760	15
WALNUTS, BLACK, CHOPPED	1 OZ	170	3
WALNUTS, ENGLISH, PIECES	1 CUP	770	22
WALNUTS, ENGLISH, PIECES	1 OZ	180	5
WATER CHESTNUTS, CANNED	1 CUP	70	17
WATERMELON, RAW	1 PIECE	155	35
WATERMELON, RAW, DICED	1 CUP	50	11
WHEAT BREAD	1 LOAF	1160	213
WHEAT BREAD	1 SLICE	65	12
WHEAT BREAD, TOASTED	1 SLICE	65	12
WHEAT FLOUR, ALL-PURPOSE,SIFTD	1 CUP	420	88
WHEAT FLOUR, ALL-PURPOSE,UNSIF	1 CUP	455	95
WHEATIES CEREAL	1 OZ	100	23
WHEAT, THIN CRACKERS	4 CRACKR	35	5
WHIPPED TOPPING, PRESSURIZED	1 CUP	155	7
WHIPPED TOPPING, PRESSURIZED	1 TBSP	10	0
WHIPPING CREAM, UNWHIPED,HEAVY	1 CUP	820	7
WHIPPING CREAM, UNWHIPED,HEAVY	1 TBSP	50	0
WHIPPING CREAM, UNWHIPED,LIGHT	1 CUP	700	7
WHIPPING CREAM, UNWHIPED,LIGHT	1 TBSP	45	0
WHITE BREAD	1 LOAF	1210	222
WHITE BREAD CRUMBS, SOFT	1 CUP	120	22

Food		Calories	Carbs
WHITE BREAD CUBES	1 CUP	80	15
WHITE BREAD, SLICE 18 PER LOAF	1 SLICE	65	12
WHITE BREAD, SLICE 22 PER LOAF	1 SLICE	55	10
WHITE BREAD, TOASTED 18 PER	1 SLICE	65	12
WHITE BREAD, TOASTED 22 PER	1 SLICE	55	10
WHITE CAKE W/ WHT FRSTNG,COMML	1 CAKE	4170	670
WHITE CAKE W/ WHT FRSTNG,COMML	1 PIECE	260	42
WHITE SAUCE W/ MILK FROM MIX	1 CUP	240	21
WHITE SAUCE, MEDIUM, HOME RECP	1 CUP	395	24
WHOLE-WHEAT BREAD	1 LOAF	1110	206
WHOLE-WHEAT BREAD	1 SLICE	70	13
WHOLE-WHEAT BREAD, TOASTED	1 SLICE	70	13
WHOLE-WHEAT FLOUR,HRD WHT,STIR	1 CUP	400	85
WHOLE-WHEAT WAFERS, CRACKERS	2 CRACKR	35	5
WINE, DESSERT	3.5 F OZ	140	8
WINE, TABLE, RED	3.5 F OZ	75	3
WINE, TABLE, WHITE	3.5 F OZ	80	3
YEAST, BAKERS, DRY, ACTIVE	1 PKG	20	3
YEAST, BREWERS, DRY	1 TBSP	25	3
YELLOW CAKE W/ CHOC FRST,FRMIX	1 CAKE	3735	638
YELLOW CAKE W/ CHOC FRST,FRMIX	1 PIECE	235	40
YELLOWCAKE W/ CHOCFRSTNG,COMML	1 CAKE	3895	620
YELLOWCAKE W/ CHOCFRSTNG,COMML	1 PIECE	245	39
YOGURT, W/ LOFAT MILK, PLAIN	8 OZ	145	16
YOGURT, W/ LOFAT MILK,FRUITFLV	8 OZ	230	43
YOGURT, W/ NONFAT MILK	8 OZ	125	17
YOGURT, W/ WHOLE MILK	8 OZ	140	11

Many of the statistics and resources for information in this book were provided by The Weight-control Information Network. (WIN) is a national service of the National Institute of Diabetes and Digestive and Kidney Diseases of the National Institutes of Health, which is the Federal Government's lead agency responsible for biomedical research on nutrition and obesity. Authorized by Congress (Public Law 103-43), WIN provides the general public, health professionals, the media, and Congress with up-to-date, science-based health information on weight control, obesity, physical activity, and related nutritional issues.

WIN answers inquiries, develops and distributes publications, and works closely with professional and patient organizations and Government agencies to coordinate resources about weight control and related issues.

Publications produced by WIN are reviewed by both NIDDK scientists and outside experts.

The text is not copyrighted. WIN encourages users of their online publications to duplicate and distribute as many copies as desired. More information can be found at

Weight-control Information Network

1 WIN WAY

BETHESDA, MD 20892-3665

Phone: (202) 828-1025

FAX: (202) 828-1028

Toll-free number: 1-877-946-4627

Internet: www.niddk.nih.gov/health/nutrit/nutrit.htm

E-mail: win@info.niddk.nih.gov

www.ingramcontent.com/pod-product-compliance
Lightning Source LLC
Chambersburg PA
CBHW020427290526
45785CB00002B/729